INTEGRATIVE MEDICINE CME
STUDY GUIDE

Accreditation Statement and Faculty Disclosure Statement:

ACCREDITATION

InnoVision Communications is accredited by the Accreditation Council for Continuing Medical Education (ACCME) to provide continuing medical education for physicians. InnoVision Communications designates these educational activities on an hour-for-hour basis toward category 1 credit of the AMA Physician's Recognition Award. Each physician should claim only those hours of credit that he/she actually spent in the educational activity.

FACULTY DISCLOSURE

All faculty participating in InnoVision Communications educational activities are expected to disclose any significant relationship with those supporting the activity or any others whose products or services are discussed.

In accordance with the Accreditation Council for Continuing Medical Education (ACCME) Standards and InnoVision Communications policy, the following faculty have indicated a relationship with the entities listed:

The following faculty intend to discuss off-label treatments:

Susan Gerik, MD
Jamal Islam, MD
Daniel Muller, MD, PhD
David Rakel, MD

The following faculty indicated no significant relationships exist:

John A. Astin, PhD	Roberta Lee, MD	Aviva Romm, AHG, CPM
James N. Dillard, MD, DC, LAC	Robert Y. Lin, MD	Robert Schiller, MD
Leo Galland, MD	Jay Lombard, DO	Edward Shalts, MD, DHT
Alan Dumoff, JD, MSW	Tieraona Low Dog, MD	Michelle Sierpina, MS
Andrea Girman, MD, MPH	Sanford Newmark, MD	Victor S. Sierpina, MD
Sezzelle Gereau Haddon, MD	Robert B. Lutz, MD, MPH	Betsy B. Singh, PhD
Susan Hadley, MD	Arya Nielsen, MA, MS, LAC,	Ellen Tattelman, MD
Randy J. Horowitz, MD, PhD	FNAAOM	Lauren Vigna, MD
Steven F. Horowitz, MD	Sunil Pai, MD	Sivarama Vinjamury,
George Kessler, DO	Francine Rainone,	MD (Ayurveda), MAON
Benjamin Kligler, MD, MPH	DO, PhD, MS	

INTEGRATIVE MEDICINE CME STUDY GUIDE

BENJAMIN KLIGLER, MD, MPH

Assistant Professor of Family Medicine
Albert Einstein College of Medicine
Bronx, New York
Research Director and Co-Director of
Integrative Medicine Fellowship
Center for Health & Healing
Beth Israel Medical Center
New York, New York

and

ROBERTA LEE, MD

Medical Director and Co-Director
Integrative Medicine Fellowship
Center for Health & Healing
Beth Israel Medical Center
New York, New York
Diplomate, Program in Integrative Medicine
University of Arizona
Tucson, Arizona

McGraw-Hill
MEDICAL PUBLISHING DIVISION

New York   Chicago   San Francisco   Lisbon   London   Madrid   Mexico City
Milan   New Delhi   San Juan   Seoul   Singapore   Sydney   Toronto

Integrative Medicine CME Study Guide

1234567890 DOC DOC 0987654

ISBN 0-07-140238-1

NOTICE

Medicine is an ever-changing science. As new research and clinical experience broaden our knowledge, changes in treatment and drug therapy are required. The authors and the publisher of this work have checked with sources believed to be reliable in their efforts to provide information that is complete and generally in accord with the standards accepted at the time of publication. However, in view of the possibility of human error or changes in medical sciences, neither the authors nor the publisher nor any other party who has been involved in the preparation or publication of this work warrants that the information contained herein is in every respect accurate or complete, and they disclaim all responsibility for any errors or omissions or for the results obtained from use of the information contained in this work. Readers are encouraged to confirm the information contained herein with other sources. For example and in particular, readers are advised to check the product information sheet included in the package of each drug they plan to administer to be certain that the information contained in this work is accurate and that changes have not been made in the recommended dose or in the contraindications for administration. This recommendation is of particular importance in connection with new or infrequently used drugs.

This book was set in Garamond by ITC.
The editors were Andrea Seils and Karen Davis.
The production supervisor was Catherine H. Saggese.
The text designer was Marsha Cohen.
RR Donnelley was printer and binder.

This book is printed on acid-free paper.

Contents

Part III

Integrative Approaches to Specific Conditions / 51

Part IV

Integrative Approaches Through the Life Cycle / 95

Part V

Legal and Ethical Issues / 121

Part VI

Current Medical Education Questions / 137

Preface

Integrative Medicine: Principles for Practice provides a comprehensive overview of the philosophy and applications of the integrative medicine approach. This accompanying *Study Guide* is designed to help readers with the process of assimilating this knowledge. Recently, many medical institutions have indicated an interest in adding examination questions on content discussed in the text and it is anticipated that soon these questions may likely be included in National Board and specialty examinations. Thus, the guide can also be helpful in preparing for test questions on this subject matter.

The first five parts of this Guide provide a set of review questions for each chapter of the text. The sixth section provides an additional set of questions with accompanying learning objectives, each corresponding to a chapter of the text, which are required for those readers planning to apply for CME credit. One credit hour per chapter is available to those readers choosing to answer these questions and submit the attached card. A total of 36 CME hours are available for those readers choosing to complete all of the CME questions in section six of the Study Guide.

Benjamin Kligler
Roberta Lee

INTEGRATIVE MEDICINE CME STUDY GUIDE

PART I

Basic Principles

CHAPTER 1
Integrative Medicine: Basic Principles

1-1. The schism of the mind–body spirit developed in 1610 is reflected initially in the writings by Descartes.

a. true
b. false

1-2. What distinguishes the basic assumptions of the holistic/integrative model from those of the reductionistic model?

a. there is no difference
b. holism asserts that the whole equals the sum of its parts but also addresses the unique properties of the whole, which behave differently
c. holism agrees with the equation that the whole equals the sum of its parts

1-3. The recognition of a health care crisis in the 1970s due to rising medical costs reflected an increase in what types of interventions that became available in biomedicine? Pick as many options as needed.

a. unique pharmaceutical agents
b. safer botanical medicines
c. a broader array of medical technologies such as, for example, laser treatments, dialysis, MRI
d. more complex surgical procedures

1-4. Integrative medicine is healing oriented. A conventional therapeutic recommendation still can be integrative if it addresses this orientation. Which of the following options are important in this approach?

a. the practitioner discusses lifestyle issues pertaining to the problem
b. the practitioner adds dietary recommendations that would possibly improve the clinical outcome
c. the practitioner discusses the diverse therapeutic options and risk–benefit ratios with the patient
d. all of the above

1-5. In an integrative interview, open-ended questions are deliberately asked. This facilitates a sense of trust and implicit invitation for the patient to share and reflect life experiences that may have contributed to the medical problem. Even though there may not be a solution, simply recognizing the pattern may be useful to the patient.

a. true
b. false

1-6. Rachel Naomi Remen, a noted medical educator and advocate for self-care in health care professionals, states that unprecedented physician burnout is evident. What options below reflect reasons that self-care proactively fights burnout?

a. it reminds us of the true meaning of our work: service

b. it gives us inner resources to face challenging clinical situations with our patients

c. it keeps us in touch with our families, our community, and our values

d. all of the above

1-7. According to Eisenberg's last survey, 70% of patients fail to mention that they use some form of alternative medicine. Some of these treatments affect medical outcomes. If the physician fails to ask about these things in taking the patient's history, the potential for "failure to diagnose" in risk management could occur.

a. true

b. false

1-8. Integrative medicine and complementary and alternative medicine (CAM) is now taught in 95% of medical schools.

a. true

b. false

1-9. Prevention is one of the major objectives in a healing-oriented practice of medicine.

a. true

b. false

1-10. It is the ultimate hope of many that integrative medicine will simply be seen as "good medicine."

a. true

b. false

CHAPTER 2

Psychosocial Determinants of Health and Illness: Reintegrating Mind, Body, and Spirit

2-1. Wilber argued for the importance of _____ but stated that _____ was detrimental.

a. differentiation; dissociation
b. reintegration; differentiation
c. defragmentation; isolation
d. dissociation; internal contemplation

2-2. The negative health effects of anxiety

a. lead to excessive sympathetic nervous system activation
b. include headache, asthma, arthritis, and ulcers
c. occur through sudden cardiac death but not myocardial infarction
d. all of the above

2-3. Benefits to mind–body approaches include which of the following:

a. minimal side effects
b. cost savings
c. improved relationships with health care providers
d. both a and b
e. all of the above

2-4. In Wilber's model, the _____ quadrant includes _____.

a. upper left; behaviors
b. lower left; concepts
c. lower right; world views
d. lower left; shared meaning

2-5. The emergence of medicine that is rooted in the physical and biological sciences is likely to have resulted from

a. the integration of the upper right and upper left quadrants
b. the integration of the upper right and lower left quadrants
c. the differentiation of the upper right and upper left quadrants
d. the differentiation of the upper right and lower left quadrants

2-6. Research examining the connection between hostility and health has statistically controlled for lifestyle risk factors, and as a result this research may

a. not be generalizable to the real world
b. be underestimating the health risks of hostility
c. not be taking those without lifestyle risk factors into consideration
d. be difficult or impossible to compare to studies of other psychosocial variables such as anxiety

2-7. Anxiety has been shown to affect which of the following systems?

a. immune
b. nervous
c. sensory
d. both a and b
e. all of the above

2-8. The belief that others are motivated by selfish concerns and are likely to be either hurtful or provoking in some way is

a. an effective defense mechanism aiding in illness prevention
b. likely to have health benefits, as long as the others are not close relatives
c. detrimental to those who rely on others for support, but not for introverts
d. none of the above
e. all of the above

2-9. Empirical evidence has shown that differences in symptom expression could be attributed to which of the following:

a. diet
b. family interactions
c. culture
d. all of the above

2-10. Research has found that unmarried individuals or persons with few social contacts were at increased risk for _____, even after statistically adjusting for _____.

a. cardiovascular death; genetic risk
b. stroke; depression
c. heart attack; socioeconomic status
d. immune deficiency disorders; age and gender

CHAPTER 3
Mind–Body Medicine

3-1. Contemporary mind–body medicine is a philosophy of care, a body of research, and an approach to therapy. It is not commonly considered to be

a. noninvasive
b. a way to promote self-reliance
c. psychotherapy
d. effective for treating pain

3-2. Increased appreciation for the therapeutic aspects of a relationship has led researchers to explore how to improve physician–patient communication. One product of such research is the concept of

a. consensual decision making
b. participatory decision making
c. physician–patient cocontracting
d. working alliance

3-3. Researchers exploring the field of psychoneuroimmunology have found that cytokines (immune products) can signal the brain directly.

a. true
b. false

3-4. The following scientist identified the "milieu interior" from which the concept of homeostasis originates:

a. Selye
b. Cannon
c. Mason
d. Bernard

3-5. Emotional inhibition (repressive coping) has been linked to lower antibody titers to Epstein–Barr virus.

a. true
b. false

3-6. Researchers claim that socioemotional experiences between mother and infant cannot influence the growth of specific postnatal brain structures.

a. true
b. false

3-7. Self-regulation, a critical way in which vital biological and behavioral responses become stabilized, begins in infancy as

a. an autoregulatory process
b. a coregulatory process
c. both

3-8. According to LeDoux's studies on the emotional circuitry of the brain, fear is learned through operant conditioning.

a. true
b. false

3-9. The brain monitors minute biological changes in the body via somatic markers, which store links between stimulus events and bodily responses. The form of memory involved in this process is

a. declarative
b. procedural
c. implicit
d. explicit

3-10. Individual response stereotypy is a term which refers to

a. cognitive attribution
b. habituated response
c. constitutional predisposition
d. all of the above

3-11. Lesions in which area of the brain have been discovered in patients who have been exposed to acute trauma?

a. hippocampus
b. hypothalamus
c. thalamus
d. cingulate gyrus

3-12. In a study of 98 primary care patients with current major depression, what percentage were not identified for a period of up to 1 year?

a. 5%
b. 15%
c. 32%
d. 48%

3-13. One of the following symptoms is *not* a key feature of posttraumatic stress disorder:

a. startle reaction
b. numbing
c. projection
d. flooding

3-14. The self in transpersonal psychology is most closely allied with

a. ego
b. personality
c. sati
d. soul

3-15. Mental healing, a psychospiritual intervention increasingly used with medical patients, encompasses the following modalities:

a. touch modalities
b. nontouch modalities
c. both touch and nontouch

3-16. Energy psychology refers to therapies that stimulate the human vibrational matrix, including meridian pathways. One such therapy, the emotional freedom technique, is known to be effective with addiction disorders, but not allergies or environment toxins.

a. true
b. false

3-17. Somatic awareness can be effective in managing chronic pain conditions, such as migraines, because it

a. directly influences bodily processes
b. heightens bodily sensitivity
c. enhances attentional focus
d. all of the above

3-18. Psychoanalysts believe that affects are first experienced as bodily feelings and that the desomatization of affects is a developmental achievement.

a. true
b. false

3-19. Brain respiration is a powerful mind–body technique associated with

a. intentional systemic mindfulness
b. vipassana
c. Zen mind
d. dahn-hak

3-20. Advanced meditators, as revealed in studies using functional MRI imagery, show increased positive affect and activation in a specific area of the brain:

a. left prefrontal cortex
b. amygdala
c. somatosensory cortex
d. anterior cingulate gyrus

CHAPTER 4
A New Definition of Patient-Centered Medicine

4-1. Ancestral healing systems differ from contemporary Western medicine in that

a. they use the placebo effect as a therapeutic tool

b. they emphasize healing the patient rather than treating the disease

c. their methods are based on predetermined principles rather than empiricism

d. they lacked the tools to perform surgical procedures

4-2. Which of the following was NOT an important aspect of Hippocratic medicine?

a. dietetics

b. environmental health

c. epidemiology of epidemics

d. magic

4-3. Randomized clinical trials

a. usually yield data that influence clinical thinking longer than data produced by clinical observation

b. often exclude patients with complex comorbidities, even though their findings will be applied to patients with complex comorbidities

c. generally recognize the difference between clinical significance and statistical significance

d. none of the above

4-4. The concept of patient-centered medicine includes the following:

a. acknowledgment of the patient's perespective.

b. a clinical vision that seeks the origins of illness and the paths to healing in the individual characteristics of each patient

c. a therapeutic approach that attempts to match treatment to the specific, sometimes idiosyncratic, requirements of each separate patient

d. all of the above

4-5. A high degree of health self-efficacy

a. often leads patients to discard effective treatment for unscientific remedies

b. is helpful for some chronic conditions but not for acute diseases

c. is enhanced by self-management education

d. none of the above

4-6. The hypothalamic–pituitary–adrenal [HPA] axis and the cytokine network

a. each form the core of separate, distinct regulatory pathways

b. work together to determine the architecture of sleep

c. are both suppressed in major depressive illness

d. need to be suppressed to cure autoimmune diseases

4-7. For the integrative practitioner, the most important feature of biochemical mediators is

a. the influence upon them of the common components of life

b. the ability of esoteric healing techniques to alter their levels

c. the ability of nutriceuticals, as opposed to drugs, to suppress them

d. none of the above

4-8. Dietary fatty acids may influence

a. prostanoid synthesis

b. peroxisome proliferator–activated receptor activity

c. response to interleukin-1.

d. all of the above

4-9. When patients are encouraged to express fully their concerns about their illnesses and their beliefs about illness

a. they are being patronized by their doctors

b. they will waste the doctor's time

c. they are likely to disagree with the doctor's appraisal, so that some form of negotiation is needed

d. they will become obsessive about illness

4-10. A person's beliefs about sickness are important because they

a. will influence symptoms and their perception

b. may increase anxiety, depression, and hopelessness

c. may interfere with the patient's ability to take an active role in his or her own care

d. all of the above

4-11. Information given to patients by physicians

a. may alleviate anxiety but never real physical symptoms

b. is inferior to the placebo effect of drug therapy

c. can decrease pain and the need for pain medication

d. is rarely cost-effective use of the physician's time

4-12. Questions about religious beliefs and spiritual practices

a. are considered intrusive by most patients

b. insult the intelligence of young patients

c. provide important prognostic information about the patient's ability to cope with disabling illness

d. waste the doctor's time

4-13. For patients with chronic headache, the best predictor of symptom relief is

a. the patient's satisfaction with the doctor's discussion of the nature of his or her problem

b. the doctor's willingness to prescribe powerful pain medication

c. the patient's desire to be pain free

d. none of the above

4-14. A study of boys with attention deficit hyperactivity disorder and a randomly selected population of schoolchildren found a correlation between low concentrations of omega-3 essential fatty acids, learning and behavior problems, and symptoms associated with essential fatty acid deficiency, which include:

a. thirst, dry skin, and dry hair
b. poor night vision
c. episodic abdominal pain
d. all of the above

4-15. Observational studies have associated variant angina, cardiac arrhythmia, migraine headache, asthma, mitral valve prolapse, chronic fatigue syndrome, attention deficit hyperactivity disorder, irritable bowel syndrome, fibromyalgia, sensorineural hearing loss, and hypertension with

a. low-fiber diets
b. magnesium deficiency or reduced magnesium intake
c. excessive consumption of seafood
d. vitamin A toxicity

4-16. Studies using experimental chambers have shown that exposure to volatile organic compounds (VOCs) at levels much lower than World Health Organization indoor air guidelines

a. are not a cause of building-related illness
b. may impair the mental function of workers who deny any adverse impact
c. can cause irritation of the respiratory system in humans and animals
d. cause brain tumors and lung cancer

4-17. Sexual abuse in childhood has been associated with

a. the development of the type A personality in men
b. an increased risk of abdominal and pelvic pain syndromes among women
c. an increase in the rate of colon and lung cancer
d. myocardial infarction and stroke in midlife

4-18. Precipitating events are

a. the real causes of disease that must be treated for healing to occur
b. figments of the patient's imagination
c. boundaries in time that separate a period of health from a period of illness
d. the main focus of conventional Western medicine

4-19. Chronic giardiasis

a. is as likely to cause constipation as diarrhea
b. may provoke asthma, urticaria, arthritis, or uveitis
c. may be undiagnosed in patients with chronic illness
d. all of the above

4-20. Controlled studies of juvenile diabetes, Graves' disease, acute appendicitis, and chronic headache reveal that

a. they are all associated with antecedent life stress
b. they respond to acupuncture and moxibustion
c. autoimmunity is a common feature of all four conditions
d. none of the above

PART II

Therapeutic Modalities

CHAPTER 5
Botanical Medicine: Overview

5-1. The actions of many botanical medicines have their roots in traditional cultures and are used in the exact manner that we use conventional pharmaceutical preparations.

a. true
b. false

5-2. Western herbalists, traditional medicine systems (e.g., Chinese medicine, East Asian medicine, Native American medicine), and biomedicine typically approach botanical use from different paradigms. Product quality and content of combinations can be accessed through several Web resources. Of the choices provided, which ones furnish such information (more than choice may be correct)?

a. Natural Medicines Comprehensive Database
b. Consumerlabs.com
c. One medicine.com
d. USP Website

5-3. The belief in whole plant products is rooted in the development of a paradigmatic divergence between alchemists and herbalists in what century?

a. Thirteenth century
b. Fourteenth century
c. Fifteenth century
d. Sixteenth century
e. Seventeenth century

5-4. Botanical substances are regulated uniformly across Europe, North and South America and Asia.

a. true
b. false

5-5. Botanical medicines in general display their clinical effects within 2 months;

a. true
b. false

5-6. Plant parts have different active constituents, and identification of these parts is crucial in quality control.

a. true
b. false

5-7. Interactions of herbal remedies and conventional prescriptions are a challenge for the physician prescriber; many available texts and online sources are readily available for reference.

a. true
b. false

5-8. Bulk products in bins are at risk of oxidizing if the turnover is low.

a. true
b. false

5-9. During the Middle Ages, Avecena, an Islamic physician, sought to preserve the knowledge of many plants used in Greek and Roman times.

a. true
b. false

5-10. One of the earliest recorded examples of clinical herbal trials is found on ancient Egyptian tablets; slaves were given many botanical substances and were observed to see what the pharmacologic effects were.

a. true
b. false

5-11. The reductionistic gold standard for research, the randomized controlled trial, is ideal for most botanical investigations, particularly formulas containing five or more different plants.

a. true
b. false

CHAPTER 6

Issues Concerning the Safety of Herbs and Phytomedicinal Preparations

6-1. In the United States, there is no formal risk–benefit assessment for botanical substances as there are for prescriptive medications because botanical medicines are considered dietary supplements under the Dietary Supplement and Health Act.

a. true
b. false

6-2. Some legal authorities looking at the ability of the FDA to enforce the safety of herbal products assert that it does have adequate authority to protect the public from unsafe herbs.

a. true
b. false

6-3. The Institute of Medicine published a proposed framework for review and public comment on evaluating the safety of dietary supplements in which year?

a. 2000
b. 2001
c. 2002
d. 2003

6-4. There are currently formal guidelines with respect to the risks of botanical supplements.

a. true
b. false

6-5. The medication colchicine comes from which of the following plants?

a. autumn crocus
b. foxglove
c. curare
d. ephedra
e. Grecian foxglove

6-6. Alkaloids are commonly found in many toxic plants.

a. true
b. false

6-7. Ephedra, or ma huang, has safely been used along with other herbs in Chinese medicine for the treatment of pulmonary conditions.

a. true
b. false

6-8. Ginger, a common kitchen spice, is discussed in the chapter under adverse effects. The German Commission E classifies ginger as unsuitable for use in pregnancy for morning sickness. A review of the literature by several researchers indicates that there is no evidence of harm to the fetus or mother with its use as an antinauseant at the dose of 1 gram of dried root.

a. true
b. false

6-9. St. John's wort interacts with two isoenzymes in the liver, CYP3A4 and CYP450. Which of the following medications are known to interact with St. John's wort because they are also metabolized in the liver?

a. cyclosporine
b. hydrochlorothiazide
c. ascorbic acid

6-10. The evidence gleaned from the Western European system currently used for pharmacovigilance demonstrates that the rate of adverse effects related to herbs and phytomedicines is significantly lower (in per capita terms) than those for conventional medications, suggesting that herbals are generally milder acting and safer than conventional drugs.

a. true
b. false

CHAPTER 7
Integrative Approach to Nutrition

7-1. The "exclusion phase" of an elimination diet protocol usually lasts

a. 7–10 days
b. 14–30 days
c. 45–60 days

7-2. During the "provocation phase" of an elimination diet, it is recommended to introduce a new food every

a. 1–2 days
b. 3–7 days
c. 7–10 days
d. 10–14 days

7-3. The glycemic index is calculated on a scale of

a. 0–10
b. 0–100
c. 0–1000

7-4. Reasonable indications for a low glycemic index diet include:

a. hyperlipidemia
b. obesity
c. diabetes
d. polycystic ovary syndrome
e. all of the above

7-5. The dietary approach to stopping hypertension (DASH) diet is specifically indicated for which of the following problems?

a. inflammatory bowel disease
b. diabetes
c. hypertension
d. chronic fatigue syndrome

7-6. When Pima Indians follow an "Anglo" diet as opposed to their traditional diet, their risk of diabetes increases by a factor of

a. 1.5
b. 2.5
c. 5.0

7-7. In general, patients with Crohn's disease are found to have a higher intake of which of the following?

a. sucrose
b. omega-6 fatty acids
c. whole grains
d. animal meats

7-8. Dietary changes that are advocated as part of the "antiinflammatory diet" include which of the following?

a. increased omega-3 fatty acids
b. decreased foods with low glycemic index
c. increased *trans* fatty acids
d. increased cruciferous vegetables

7-9. The standard American diet has an omega-6 essential fatty acid/omega-3 essential fatty acid ratio of roughly

a. 2:1
b. 4:1
c. 10:1
d. 20:1

7-10. Animals fed grasses rich in omega-3 essential fatty acids (EFAs) produce meat lower in omega-3 than animals fed sources rich in omega-6 EFAs.

a. true
b. false

7-11. One of the effects of increased insulin is the upregulation of delta-5-desaturase, an important enzyme in fatty acid metabolism. This leads to which of the following:

a. increased dihomo-gamma-linoleic acid (DGLA) synthesis
b. increased arachidonic acid synthesis
c. increase in inflammation
d. increase in breakdown of arachidonic acid

7-12. The following grains should definitely be excluded from a gluten-free diet:

a. wheat
b. barley
c. rice
d. quinoa
e. buckwheat

7-13. The following should all be eliminated if a soy-free diet is being recommended:

a. hydrolyzed plant protein
b. peanut oil
c. soybean oil
d. modified food starch
e. natural flavoring

7-14. Patients with untreated celiac disease may be at a significantly increased risk for development of certain gastrointestinal cancers.

a. true
b. false

CHAPTER 8
Chiropractic and Osteopathic Care

8-1. Chiropractic was founded in America and osteopathy was founded in Europe.

a. true
b. false

8-2. Chiropractic developed out of an historical context when vitalistic health philosophies were emerging in contrast to the heroic medicine of the post–Civil War era.

a. true
b. false

8-3. The most current research shows chiropractic care to be effective for migraine, cervicogenic, and tension headaches.

a. true
b. false

8-4. Chiropractic adjustment may help some patients with respiratory conditions like chronic obstructive pulmonary disease and asthma through its effect on the autonomic nervous system.

a. true
b. false

8-5. Chiropractic care for patients with recurrent otitis media is effective for all of the following reasons EXCEPT:

a. it increases lymphatic drainage
b. it helps drain eustachian tubes, which are horizontal in young children
c. it helps decrease inflammation
d. it decreases food allergies

8-6. To be licensed, chiropractors have to pass rigorous written and practical board exams.

a. true
b. false

8-7. There is evidence in the literature that chiropractic might cure all of the following conditions EXCEPT:

a. duodenal ulcer
b. acute low back pain
c. cancer
d. headache

8-8. The National Institutes of Health started to fund chiropractic research in the 1990s.

a. true
b. false

8-9. Chiropractic care is included in which of the following programs:

a. Medicare
b. Department of Defense and Veterans Administration
c. most HMOs
d. state disability programs
e. all of the above

8-10. Osteopathy involves joint and soft tissue manipulation.

a. true
b. false

8-11. Some osteopathic techniques involve manipulation of the viscera.

a. true
b. false

8-12. Osteopaths are licensed to write prescriptions and perform surgery.

a. true
b. false

8-13. One commonality between chiropractic and osteopathy is the focus on the relationship between structure and function of the human body.

a. true
b. false

8-14. Both chiropractic and osteopathy utilize cranial adjusting techniques.

a. true
b. false

8-15. Research on osteopathy has suggested effectiveness for the following conditions:

a. pneumonia
b. cholecystectomy
c. influenza
d. acute low back pain
e. all of the above

8-16. Research shows a positive effect of osteopathy and chiropractic on the length of labor.

a. true
b. false

8-17. Chiropractic adjustments are specific to a particular vertebra and a particular direction of motion, whereas mobilization techniques restore movement to a general area of the body.

a. true
b. false

8-18. Postgraduate chiropractic education such as continuing medical education courses are required by many states in the United States.

a. true
b. false

8-19. Doctors of chiropractic can receive postdoctoral "diplomates" in various specialties such as orthopedics, sports injuries, nutrition, and pediatrics.

a. true
b. false

8-20. Visceral manipulation might be effective for the following conditions:

a. dysmenorrhea
b. gastroesophageal reflux disease
c. irritable bowel syndrome
d. incontinence
e. all of the above

CHAPTER 9

Acupuncture and East Asian Medicine

9-1. Bloodletting is a practice formerly done in acupuncture, but now no longer a part of acupuncture practice.

a. true
b. false

9-2. Professional acupuncture training leading to licensure requires at least

a. 400 hours of training
b. 1750 hours of training
c. 3000 hours of training

9-3. Studies since 1997 on the use of acupuncture for stroke rehabilitation seem to indicate that acupuncture is not as helpful for this condition as was originally thought.

a. true
b. false

9-4. Generally speaking, studies since 1997 have demonstrated a greater benefit of acupuncture when it has been compared to which of the following:

a. invasive sham needling
b. noninvasive sham needling
c. transcutaneous electrical nerve stimulation (TENS) treatment

9-5. Regarding substance abuse treatment, studies since 1998 have found some positive results for acupuncture treatment in which of the following conditions?

a. alcohol abuse
b. cocaine abuse
c. smoking cessation

9-6. Studies since 1998 have moved acupuncture for the treatment of fibromyalgia from the "may be helpful" category to the "promising" category.

a. true
b. false

9-7.   The radial pulse on the right wrist nearest the wrist crease is associated with the

a. lungs
b. heart
c. spleen
d. kidney

9-8.   Heat generally

a. rises in the body
b. is associated with redness
c. increases the pulse rate
d. all of the above

9-9.   Dampness

a. pours down
b. winds up
c. moves laterally in the channels
d. inverts interstitially

9-10.   The heart and spleen are coupled with which organs?

a. small intestine and stomach
b. pericardium and stomach
c. liver and lungs
d. kidney and bladder

9-11.   Studies show that acupuncture can

a. treat nausea
b. prevent recurrence of urinary tract infections
c. reduce the length of the initial stage of labor
d. all of the above

9-12.   Each of the organs in East Asian medicine has a similar organ in the West, except for the

a. San Jiao
b. Li
c. Bu tong
d. Sha

9-13.   Acupuncture was likely derived from the practice of therapeutic

a. bloodletting
b. lancing
c. cautery
d. all of the above

9-14.   Acupuncture was first referred to in a Chinese text written in

a. 90 BC
b. 165 BC
c. 200 BC
d. 200 AD

9-15.   Most of the main acupuncture points are found at

a. intramuscular connective tissue planes
b. exact distances from the heart
c. sites proximal to nerve ganglia
d. crossing of blood vessels

9-16.   Chinese medicine classic texts correspond in large part to the

a. Hippocratic Corpus
b. Ebers Papyrus
c. Talmud
d. none of the above

9-17.   How many licensed acupuncturists are practicing in the U.S.?

a. 10–15000
b. 6–8000
c. 100,000
d. 2000

9-18.   Physician courses of acupuncture study are typically

a. 300 hours
b. 450 hours
c. 600 hours
d. 4500 hours

9-19.   Gua sha and cupping are techniques that remove

a. blood stasis
b. shedding epidermal layers
c. pooling edema
d. wind from the channels

9-20.   Moxibustion burns fibers from the plant

a. *Artemesia vulgaris*
b. *Angelica sinensis*
c. *Poria cocos*
d. *Ma huang*

9-21.   The central focus of traditional East Asian medical assessment is

a. the patient's experience of their problem
b. the pulse
c. the tongue
d. palpation

CHAPTER 10
Ayurvedic Medicine

10-1. Ayurveda incorporates the following four into one meaningful system:

a. body (sarira), mind (indriya), senses (satva), soul (atma)

b. body (sarira), mind (indriya), senses, (satva), knowledge (veda)

c. body (sarira), mind (indriya), life (ayus), soul (atma)

d. body (sarira), life knowledge (ayurveda), senses (satva), soul (atma)

10-2. The "father of plastic surgery" is

a. Charak

b. Sushruta

c. Asthanga

d. Kashyapa

10-3. Which of the following is not among the three major treatises or texts?

a. *Charaka Samhita*

b. *Sushruta Samhita*

c. *Astanga Hridaya*

d. *Bhela Samhita*

10-4. According to Ayurveda, these are the four goals of life:

a. virtue (dharma), wealth (artha), enjoyment (kama), life (ayus)

b. virtue (dharma), wealth (artha), knowledge (veda), salvation (moksha)

c. virtue (dharma), body (sarira), enjoyment (kama), salvation (moksha)

d. virtue (dharma), wealth (artha), enjoyment (kama), salvation (moksha)

10-5. The following are the five basic elements (Panch Maha Bhuta) in Ayurveda:

a. earth (prithivi), water (jala), fire (teja), body (sarira), space (akasha)

b. earth (prithivi), water (jala), senses (satva), air (vayu), space (akasha)

c. earth (prithivi), soul (atma), fire (teja), air (vayu), space (akasha)

d. earth (prithivi), water (jala), fire (teja), air (vayu), space (akasha)

10-6. Which of the following three are known as doshas?

a. Vata, Dhatu, Kapha

b. Vata, Mala, Kapha

c. Vata, Atma, Kapha

d. Vata, Pitta, Kapha

10-7.   The structure of the body is formed by the

a. Dhatus
b. Mala
c. Doshas
d. Vata

10-8.   Prakriti is defined as

a. structure of the body
b. metabolic waste
c. one's individual constitution
d. digestive strength

10-9.   Pitta dosha is maximum during which stage of life?

a. childhood
b. middle age
c. old age
d. throughout one's life

10-10.   Which of the following is not one of the Saptadhatus?

a. Rasa
b. Rakta
c. Mamsa
d. Mala

10-11.   Which refers to the "communication channels"?

a. Dosa
b. Dhatu
c. Sroctas
d. Mala

10-12.   The build-up of toxins and waste in the body is referred to as

a. Agni
b. Ama
c. Akasha
d. Artha

10-13.   Which of the following are the fundamental properties of the mind?

a. Sattva, rajas, and tamas
b. Vata, pitta and kapha
c. Dosha, dhatu, and mala
d. Sarira and atma

10-14.   This is the number of tastes according to Ayurveda:

a. Four
b. Six
c. Five
d. Three

10-15.   Hatha yoga incorporates the following things:

a. asanas (postures)
b. breath work (pranayama)
c. meditation
d. all of the above

10-16.   One of the most common types of oil massage is called

a. vamana
b. abhyanga
c. nasya
d. virecana

10-17.   The Virecana procedure is best to eliminate this Dosa:

a. Vata
b. Pitta
c. Kapha
d. Rakta

10-18.   The following procedure is the treatment choice in Vata disorders:

a. Vamana
b. Virecana
c. Basti
d. Raktamoksana

10-19. The predominant involvement of this Dhatu is seen in Sthoulya Roga:

a. Rasa
b. Rakta
c. Mamsa
d. Meda

10-20. The following is analogous to atherosclerosis in Ayurveda:

a. meda
b. margavarana
c. mala
d. moksha

CHAPTER 11
Movement and Body-Centered Therapies

11-1. Qigong is translated as

a. Qi exercise
b. movement therapy
c. shadow boxing
d. breath of life

11-2. The function of Qi is to

a. hold organs in place
b. warm the body
c. protect the body against disease
d. all of the above

11-3. One group of hypertensive patients was treated with antihypertensive medication only and another group of hypertensive patients took medication and practiced qigong 30 minutes twice a day. The qigong group vs the medication-only group had the following incidence of stroke:

a. 20.5% vs 40.7%
b. 25.5% vs 45.3%
c. 37.7% vs 61.1%
d. 45.2% vs 27.4%

11-4. Postnatal Qi is derived

a. from food, liquids, and lifestyle
b. from the parents
c. during conception
d. from the kidneys

11-5. The blood chemistry of hypertensive patients shows improvement with qigong exercises in

a. plasma coagulation fibrinolysis
b. blood viscosity
c. plasminogen activator inhibitor
d. all of the above

11-6. Movement therapies in alternative medicine involve active participation of the patient and a physical interaction between the provider and patient.

a. true
b. false

11-7. References to the postures of Hatha yoga include:
1. the 6th century BC Upanishads
2. the *Yoga Sutras* by Patanjali in BC
3. the *Hatha Yoga Pradipika* by Swatmarama
4. *Hatharatnavali* by Srinivasabhatta Mahayogindra

a. 1 is correct
b. 1 and 3 are correct
c. 4 is correct
d. all are correct

11-8. Asanas or postures, breathing or pranayama, and meditation are all commonly part of Hatha yoga.

a. true
b. false

11-9. Which of the following yoga teachers were not students of the Hatha yoga master Sri T. Krishnamacharya?

a. B.K.S. Iyengar
b. Pattabhi Jois
c. T.K.V. Desikachar
d. Bikram Choudry

11-10. One of the main theories on the possible mechanisms of action of Hatha yoga is that it can be used to reset the resting tone of the autonomic nervous system.

a. true
b. false

11-11. The styles of meditation that have been specifically studied for their health benefits are
1. mindfulness-based stress reduction
2. Vipassana meditation
3. transcendental meditation
4. Siddha yoga meditation

a. 1 only
b. 1 and 3
c. 1, 2, and 3
d. all of the above

11-12. Rolfing is a manual medicine therapy that
1. was initially developed as an adjunct to orthopedic medicine
2. involves direct pressure to trigger points located on meridians
3. focuses on treatment of the connective tissue fascia
4. began in Sweden in the 1920s

a. 1 is true
b. 1 and 3 are true
c. 1, 2, and 3 are true
d. all are true

11-13. Therapeutic massage involves manipulation of the soft tissue structure of the body.

a. true
b. false

11-14. Commonly used techniques used in therapeutic massage include:
1. friction
2. effleurage
3. petrissage
4. vibration/percussion

a. 1 is true
b. 1 and 3 are true
c. 1, 2, and 3 are true
d. all are true

11-15. Petrissage refers to the technique of kneading the muscles that is used to increase circulation to the muscle bed.

a. true
b. false

11-16. Meditation practices, regardless of the style, have several features in common, including:
1. sessions usually last at least 15–20 minutes, and may last much longer
2. attention is often focused on the breath or a mantra
3. it may be useful in reducing stress

a. 1 is true
b. 1 and 3 are true
c. 1, 2, and 3 are true
d. all are true

11-17. Pranayama is considered to be the "yogic science of breath control," and preliminary evidence has shown that it may be useful as an adjunctive therapy for the treatment of asthma.

a. true
b. false

11-18. A series of clinical studies have been done on the use of yoga and pranayama for
1. asthma
2. headaches
3. hypertension
4. low back pain

a. 1 is true
b. 1, 2, and 3 are true
c. 4 is true
d. all are true

11-19. Medical qigong is divided into two parts: internal and external. Internal Qi is developed by individual practice of qigong exercises. When qigong practitioners become sufficiently skilled, they can use external Qi (*waiqi* in Chinese) to "emit" Qi for the purpose of healing another person.

a. true
b. false

11-20. Clinical trials in Hatha yoga include its use in a variety of areas including:
1. osteoarthritis
2. carpal tunnel syndrome
3. high blood pressure
4. headaches

a. 1 is true
b. 2 is true
c. 3 is true
d. all are true

11-21. Commonly available therapeutic massages include:
1. deep tissue massage, which releases tension and increases relaxation through massage of the superficial and deep muscles
2. sports massage to enhance athletic performance and increase the rate of recovery
3. connective tissue massage, using light and deep massage of the superficial and deep connective tissues to stimulate the neural reflex arcs connecting the musculoskeletal system and the internal organs
4. trigger point massage and shiatsu massage, involving deep finger pressure on trigger points or acupressure points

a. 1 is true
b. 2 is true
c. 1 and 3 are true
d. all are true

CHAPTER 12
Homeopathy

12-1. Homeopathy was developed by

a. Hippocrates
b. Hahnemann
c. Herring
d. Hemingway

12-2. Homeopathy was discovered and developed as the result of

a. channeling of information
b. traditional Indian medicine
c. translation of Arabic, Ancient Greek, and Latin texts
d. experimental work

12-3. Clinical research data on homeopathy

a. do not exist
b. clearly show that homeopathic remedies are not different from placebo
c. are mixed, showing a trend of homeopathy to be different from placebo
d. are not necessary because homeopathic remedies do not work

12-4. Homeopathic remedies are prepared by

a. patients according to instructions given by homeopaths
b. by homeopathic practitioners
c. in specialized homeopathic pharmacies according to strict standards of the Homeopathic Pharmacopoeia of the United States and regulated by the FDA
d. major pharmaceutical companies

12-5. Homeopathic concentration 30X means that the substance was diluted

a. 30 times
b. 10^{-3} times
c. 10^{-30} times
d. 10^{-60} times

12-6. Homeopathic remedies

a. can be taken many times a day without any harm
b. must be administered 8 pellets at a time on a TID schedule
c. may cause a worsening of the target condition if repeated too frequently

12-7. In his writings, Samuel Hahnemann

a. spoke against polypharmacy and barbaric methods of treatment, and promoted differential therapeutics and an experimental approach to finding new medications
b. condemned biological science and approved theories of signatures, phlebotomy, and polypharmacy
c. translated works of ancient physicians

12-8. The initial homeopathic evaluation

a. is done through palpation and laboratory work
b. is done by electronic devices connected to the patient
c. consists of a general medical examination and the standard organ/system review, with the emphasis on the unique characteristics of the patient
d. consists of a general medical examination and the standard organ/system review, with the emphasis on specific laboratory data characteristic to the pathological process in question

12-9. External *Arnica* preparations

a. should never be used
b. should never be placed on broken skin
c. should never be used for minor bruises
d. should always accompany the internal administration of *Arnica*

12-10. *Bellis perennis* is frequently indicated for

a. abdominal or/and pelvic trauma
b. abdominal surgery
c. both
d. neither

12-11. A remedy known to be helpful in a large percentage of cases of right-sided deltoid pain and/or right shoulder arthritis is

a. *Bryonia*
b. *Arnica*
c. *Sanguinaria*
d. *Hypericum*

12-12. *Spongia tosta*

a. is the most frequently indicated remedy in treatment of croup after the first 24 hours of the illness
b. is indicated when the patient feels better from drinking warm liquids or eating warm food
c. is indicated when the patient feels better from bending the head forward
d. all of the above

12-13. *Hepar sulphuris* is indicated when the patient suffering from croup is

a. very quiet and pleasant
b. much better from being uncovered and cold
c. better from throwing the head backward
d. all of the above

12-14. *Anas barbariae hepatis et cordis extractum 200C*

a. is produced under the brand names Occilococcinum and Flu Solution
b. has been evaluated in double-blind placebo-controlled studies with promising results
c. is efficacious in the treatment of early stages of the flu and common cold
d. all of the above

12-15. Patients with flu or a common cold may benefit from *Arsenicum album* if they present with

a. gastrointestinal complaints
b. significant anxiety with fear of dying and a desire for company
c. a thirst for small sips of water
d. all of the above

12-16. Patients with the flu or a common cold may benefit from *Bryonia* if they present with

a. a desire to be absolutely still
b. sudden onset of the illness
c. lack of muscular pains and aches
d. all of the above

12-17.   Patients with the flu or a common cold may benefit from *Baptisia tinctoria* if they present with the main complaint of

a. severe, unbearable aching
b. a thirst for cold drinks despite feeling chilly
c. a delusion that their body is broken into pieces or double
d. aggravation at 10 AM

12-18.   Patients with the flu or a common cold may benefit from *Gelsemium* if they present with main complaints of

a. marked debility
b. a sensation of heaviness of head and droopy eyelids
c. minimal thirst
d. all of the above

12-19.   Children with acute otitis media may benefit from *Pulsatilla* if they present with one or more of the following symptoms:

a. the child is weepy, needs affection, and wants to be carried slowly and tenderly
b. the illness begins with a cold, frequently with thick green or yellow nasal discharge that develops into otitis media
c. a changeable condition: one moment the child is very sick, the next moment playing, looking much improved
d. no thirst and pale face despite high fever
e. all of the above

12-20.   Children with acute otitis media may benefit from *Chamomilla* if they present with one or more of the following symptoms:

a. the child is unbearably irritable, screaming, and demanding and wants to be carried at all times
b. painless otitis
c. the child is irritable, but better by staying in a quiet, dark room
d. all of the above

CHAPTER 13

Physical Activity and Exercise

13-1. There is good evidence to support the recommendation that all individuals should be regularly physically active.

a. true
b. false

13-2. Physical inactivity has been identified as an independent risk factor for cardiovascular disease.

a. true
b. false

13-3. Historically, a significant majority of exercise research focused solely on the cardiovascular benefits of aerobic activity.

a. true
b. false

13-4. Researchers have been challenged to identify a dose–response relationship between exercise and cardiovascular fitness.

a. true
b. false

13-5. Performing ~30 minutes of moderate-intensity activity consumes approximately 300 kcal of energy.

a. true
b. false

13-6. Youth demonstrate significant decreases in overall physical activity around the time of adolescence.

a. true
b. false

13-7. Young people should not engage in strength/resistance training until they are of high school age.

a. true
b. false

13-8. A balanced activity program for seniors should encourage cardiorespiratory, resistance, and flexibility exercises.

a. true
b. false

13-9. Tai Chi has been shown to provide significant benefits for seniors, including the frail elderly.

a. true
b. false

13-10. Physical inactivity and poor nutritional choices have been identified as leading causes of morbidity and mortality.

a. true
b. false

13-11. There is evidence to support the role of physical activity in all levels of disease prevention.

a. true
b. false

13-12. As currently defined, lifestyle activities include those activities consistent with active living, such as walking to the grocery store and using a push-type lawn mower.

a. true
b. false

13-13. Integrative approaches should seek to make physical activity and exercise a natural part of everyday living rather than solely a health-related requirement.

a. true
b. false

13-14. Research has suggested that the optimal time for building bone density in women is during the late teen years and early 20s.

a. true
b. false

13-15. Exercise and physical activity are terms that may be used interchangeably.

a. true
b. false

13-16. Fundamental to integrative approaches to physical activity and exercise is role modeling on the part of the health care practitioner.

a. true
b. false

CHAPTER 14
Spirituality and Health

14-1. Traditional healing practices have been intrinsically and immutably interwoven with

a. music and dancing
b. spiritual practice
c. phases of the moon
d. none of these

14-2. The vocabulary of traditional Chinese medicine does not differentiate spiritual and mental healing from physical healing. Rather, these represent

a. ancient Chinese deities
b. five elements of ancestor worship
c. unknown elements of the world
d. different levels of healing in a holistic continuum

14-3. One model freed science from explaining existential issues. It was

a. Taoism
b. Freudian
c. Judeo-Christian
d. Cartesian

14-4. The disconnect between spirituality and mind–body is not addressed by

a. popular culture and contemporary literature
b. contemporary scientific quest for knowledge
c. religious communities
d. psychoneuroimmunology

14-5. Medical students tend best to comprehend the definitions of organized religion and personal spirituality when the professor

a. shares the same religion as the medical student
b. allows students to draw their own conclusions whatever they may be
c. draws a parallel between the student's "personal spirituality" and the organized religious practices to which many of them have been exposed while growing up
d. presents the evidence revealed in the epidemiology of religion studies

14-6. Studies on the epidemiology of health and religion have generally focused on

a. plants and animals
b. foreign countries instead of the United States
c. religious practice, with attendance as a measurable variable
d. all of the above

14-7. Ninety-one medical schools address such topics in training programs because

a. there is a federal law requiring inclusion of such topics
b. it creates one more hurdle to successful graduation
c. there is insufficient material to cover in the 4 years of medical school
d. they help students understand the cultural aspects of the practice of medicine

14-8. Based on their own belief system, persons within some religious groups find it proper to fight for every last breath of life no matter how intricate and complex the medical intervention.

a. true
b. false

14-9. Some persons have religious belief systems that make them able to accept peacefully an end-of-life transition with minimal medical heroics.

a. true
b. false

14-10. While not every patient need be queried about spirituality in a longitudinal, continuity-of-care type of therapeutic relationship,

a. physicians should ask these questions quarterly
b. often spiritual issues will emerge spontaneously and organically
c. physicians have no interest in spiritual beliefs of their patients
d. patients no longer feel the need to communicate deep personal information with their physicians

14-11. A skilled clinician may use Maslow's hierarchy of needs

a. as a guide in assessing patient readiness and the appropriateness of discussing spiritual matters
b. as a scientific tool for cataloguing patient demographics
c. for scientific study of patients on Medicaid
d. none of the above

14-12. Several studies have shown that patients would like to discuss such spiritual matters with their physicians, and even

a. ask their physicians to join their faith community
b. have the physician join them in prayer
c. write long personal letters to their physicians about spiritual beliefs
d. convert to the faith of the physician

14-13. At this author's medical school, faculty provide their students with vocabulary and domains of inquiry which

a. influence students' future religious behavior and practices
b. help students elicit a spiritual history in a comfortable manner
c. understand that spiritual history is irrelevant to the patient's plan of care
d. all of the above

14-14. Researchers have widely studied and reported the direct effects of prayer and positive intentionality on

a. people and animals
b. microbes
c. random number generators
d. all of these

14-15. One chaplain published a view that incorporating spiritual matters into health care

a. can trivialize religion by subsuming it into medical treatment as just another modality
b. can cause physical harm to patients
c. can diminish the physician's effectiveness in patient care
d. none of the above

14-16. Some people believe that only clinical trials rather than epidemiologic studies on church attendance data are likely to be definitive in defining the effect of religion on health.

a. true
b. false

14-17. In the controversy surrounding faith and religion as adjunctive to medical treatments, some critics believe

a. it is a sin against God for the two to intersect
b. it is premature to promote integrating the two
c. it is not happening in US health care, so the discussion is irrelevant
d. technology has greatly reduced the role of religion in health care

14-18. Scholars are now taking seriously the potential of prayer to influence health outcomes, and a large number of prayer studies have been designed and executed, many with statistically significant outcomes.

a. true
b. false

14-19. That certain repeatable EEG patterns can be identified during prayer and meditation suggests that the proximal cause of consciousness of the Divine is mediated through

a. our central nervous systems
b. solar flares
c. extended periods of sleeplessness
d. epileptic episodes

14-20. Healing is defined as "making whole." The author concludes that attaining a view of Oneness that is mystical and transcendent is

a. unattainable in today's health care arena
b. the ultimate state in which healing may flourish
c. something best left to the mystics and priests
d. a variety of religious experience only remotely related to health and well-being

CHAPTER 15
Informatics and Integrative Medicine

15-1. For coverage of manual medicine, a good database to search is

a. HealthStar
b. CINAHL
c. CARDS
d. Napralert

15-2. Keyword searches are best used when

a. you do not know the MeSH heading
b. there are a large number of articles on your topic
c. there is no MeSH heading for your topic

15-3. It is helpful to use subheadings in a MEDLINE search

a. for all your searches
b. when you are looking for a specific aspect of your topic
c. when your retrieval is small

15-4. Subscription databases primarily differ from bibliographic databases by providing full text information on health conditions, treatments, and drug and/or herbal monographs.

a. true
b. false

15-5. A Website that provides systematic reviews on pain and anesthesia is

a. Pain Link
b. CAMPAIN
c. Pain Research at Oxford

15-6. Exploding the term *Medicine, Traditional* will retrieve articles on all major indigenous healing systems.

a. true
b. false

15-7. When combining search terms using the Boolean operator *AND*, you are

a. narrowing your search
b. expanding your search

15-8. It is advisable to use as many relevant synonyms as possible when doing a search.

a. true
b. false

15-9. It is important to use truncation when doing a keyword search.

a. true
b. false

15-10. When searching herbal medicine in MEDLINE, it is a good idea to include the names of plant constituents in addition to the plant name.

a. true
b. false

15-11. Cross-cultural medicine can be effectively searched in the following databases except

a. CINAHL
b. MEDLINE
c. Cochrane Library
d. HomInform

CHAPTER 16
Selected Issues in Environmental Medicine

16-1. Under the Clean Water Act, the US EPA sets water quality standards for all contaminants found in groundwater.

a. true
b. false

16-2. The Safe Drinking Water Act was first passed in 1974, and has been amended twice since then (in 1986 and 1996). The SDWA mandates the USEPA to do which of the following?

a. set and enforce national health-based quality standards for naturally occurring and man-made compounds found in tap water
b. regulate discharges made to surface water sources
c. monitor the patency of public water systems infrastructure
d. increase public access to information about drinking water

16-3. Enforceable pollutant standards for tap water include which of the following?

a. maximum contaminant goal levels (MCGLs)
b. total dissolved solids (TDS)
c. maximum contaminant levels (MCLs)
d. all of the above

16-4. As much as 45% of gastrointestinal illness may be due to consumption of drinking water currently meeting federal water quality standards.

a. true
b. false

16-5. Infectious agents responsible for dermatitis associated with recreational water contamination include all of the following except

a. *Shigella* spp.
b. *Legionella*
c. *Campylobacter*
d. *Pseudomonas* spp.

16-6. *Cryptosporidium* is considered a significant threat to the US water supply. Factors that make this organism a health concern include:

a. high level of infectivity
b. resistance to chlorine disinfection
c. both
d. neither

16-7. According to a 2002 CDC report, infectious agents causing the majority of groundwater outbreaks were found in community wells not regulated by the US EPA.

a. true
b. false

16-8. By-products of the water disinfection process have been linked to adverse health effects. These include all of the following except

a. breast cancer
b. neural tube defects
c. spontaneous abortion
d. lung cancer

16-9. The upper intake level (UIL) for fluoride is

a. 8 mg daily
b. 5 mg daily
c. 10 mg daily
d. 3 mg daily

16-10. The only emission monitored by the EPA which has increased since 1970 is

a. particulate matter
b. carbon monoxide
c. nitrogen oxides
d. sulfur dioxide

16-11. Antioxidants that have been shown in the literature to be helpful against air pollution include:

a. vitamin C
b. selenium
c. vitamin E
d. beta carotene
e. garlic

16-12. An organized environmental history-taking includes which of the following points?

a. surgeries
b. home
c. hobbies
d. occupation
e. toxic chemical checklist
f. diet

16-13. Building-related illness (BRI) and sick building syndrome (SBS) are the same condition.

a. true
b. false

PART III

Integrative Approaches to Specific Conditions

CHAPTER 17
Integrative Approach to Allergy

17-1. What medication has some reported success in chronic idiopathic urticaria patients who failed to respond to conventional medications?

a. digoxin
b. thyroxine
c. nifedipine
d. calcium

17-2. Which of the following is not a recommended component of the evaluation of cold urticaria?

a. cold agglutinins
b. cryoglobulins
c. syphilis
d. Lyme titer

17-3. In chronic urticaria, conventional treatments often result in complete resolution of disease.

a. true
b. False

17-4. In chronic urticaria, which of the following combinations are acceptable regimens?

a. loratadine + hydroxyzine
b. cetirizine + diphenhydramine
c. loratadine + ranitidine
d. diphenhydramine + cimetidine

17-5. Which of the following agents has not been specifically recommended for amelioration of symptoms of chronic urticaria?

a. leukotriene antagonists
b. doxepin
c. ketotifen
d. thyroxine
e. lamivudine

17-6. Oral corticosteroids are often the ideal choice for the treatment of chronic urticaria.

a. true
b. false

17-7. Patients with chronic urticaria frequently benefit from prescription antifungals.

a. true
b. false

17-8. An elimination diet is a reasonable first step in treating chronic urticaria.

a. true
b. false

17-9. Allergic conjunctivitis is often accompanied by allergic rhinitis.

a. true
b. false

17-10. Which of the following medications have both H_1-receptor blocking and mast cell stabilizing effects?

a. nedocromil
b. naphazoline
c. lodoxamide
d. polysporin

17-11. Ketorolac is FDA approved for treatment of allergic conjunctivitis.

a. true
b. false

17-12. The addition of systemic antihistamines is not usually effective in patients who do not respond to nonsteroid antiallergic ophthalmics.

a. true
b. false

17-13. Which of the following statements are true?

a. corticosteroid ophthalmics are essential for patients with allergic conjunctivitis that do not respond to other medications
b. prior to initiating treatment with an ocular steroid preparation, care must be exercised to be sure of the correct diagnosis
c. all corticosteroid preparations can potentially raise intraocular pressure in susceptible individuals, but this rise is usually transient
d. corticosteroid ophthalmics can be used with impunity

17-14. Food allergies that begin in late childhood or adulthood will persist unless complete avoidance of the offending allergen from the diet is achieved.

a. true
b. false

17-15. Tolerance to an allergen will usually occur within 2 years of an appropriate elimination diet.

a. true
b. false

17-16. Like the skin test, a negative RAST is not useful in excluding a presumed allergen.

a. true
b. false

17-17. The gold standard of food sensitivity tests is the double-blind placebo-controlled food challenge.

a. true
b. false

17-18. All allergic individuals with a history of anaphylactic reactions should carry an epinephrine self-injector (such as Epi-Pen) to use in the event of accidental exposure.

a. true
b. false

17-19. Autoimmune disorders, constipation, gastroesophageal reflux disease, and even nephropathy have been associated with ingestion of cow's milk in susceptible individuals.

a. true
b. false

17-20. The elimination diet is continued for at least 8–10 days.

a. true
b. false

17-21.   Licorice has antispasmodic, anti-inflammatory, expectorant, laxative, and soothing properties.

a. true
b. false

17-22.   Quercetin is a potent antioxidant, and has been shown to be useful in inhibiting allergic disease mechanisms.

a. true
b. false

CHAPTER 18
Integrative Approach to Cardiovascular Health

18-1. Breast cancer kills twice as many women as heart disease.

a. true
b. false

18-2. Coronary artery disease incidence is primarily determined by

a. heredity
b. acquired risk factors

18-3. Death rates from coronary artery disease vary throughout the world but are consistent across the United States.

a. true
b. false

18-4. Alternative and complementary approaches to coronary artery disease should play an important role in the treatment of unstable angina pectoris.

a. true
b. false

18-5. Based on current data, which of the following is likely to be most effective in preventing recurrence after a myocardial infarction?

a. medical therapy
b. lifestyle intervention
c. angioplasty/stenting
d. a + b
e. a + c

18-6. Improvement in stress myocardial perfusion imaging as demonstrated by serial positron emission tomography (PET) while encouraging, does not correlate with improved outcome.

a. true
b. false

18-7. The American Heart Association diets (stages I and II) have been shown to positively affect which of the following outcomes:

a. coronary artery disease progression
b. cardiac event rates
c. both
d. neither

18-8. The protective effect of the specific fats emphasized in the Lyon Heart Study appears to be mediated via a change in which of the following?

a. total cholesterol
b. alpha-lipoprotein a
c. LDL-C
d. all of the above
e. none of the above

18-9. Very-low-fat vegetarian diets (less than 10% total fat) have not been shown to be valuable for the treatment of coronary artery disease.

a. true
b. false

18-10. In observational studies, vegetarianism is associated with lower rates of coronary disease.

a. true
b. false

18-11. Simple carbohydrates and other high–glycemic-index foods are believed to increase the risk of coronary disease by which mechanism?

a. raising the total cholesterol
b. promoting insulin resistance
c. interfering with absorption of healthy fats

18-12. People who can perform only a minimal amount of exercise on a diagnostic treadmill test, with or without known coronary disease, have a significantly higher risk of which of the following?

a. cardiovascular mortality
b. all-cause mortality
c. both

18-13. With appropriate support, dieting alone is usually enough to maintain weight loss, even without an exercise program.

a. true
b. false

18-14. The incidence of sedentary lifestyle in the United States in recent years has been

a. increasing
b. decreasing

18-15. Long-distance running has been shown to have a benefit in cardiovascular disease superior to that of a regular walking program.

a. true
b. false

18-16. The risk of death at rest is higher than that during exercise.

a. true
b. false

18-17. Common clinical markers of increased coronary risk include

a. increased waist size
b. high triglycerides
c. both
d. neither

18-18. The level of alcohol that appears to provide the maximum benefit in terms of cardiovascular risk and all-cause mortality appears to be

a. 2 drinks per day
b. 2–4 drinks per week
c. 6–8 drinks per week

18-19. Both type A (aggressiveness, hostility, and time urgency) and type D (social isolation, anxiety, and depression) personalities are at increased coronary disease risk.

a. true
b. false

18-20. Large doses of which of the following have been shown to improve outcome in coronary disease?

a. coenzyme Q10
b. vitamin E
c. beta-carotene
d. all of the above
e. none of the above

CHAPTER 19
Integrative Approach to Chronic Fatigue Syndrome

19-1. The etiology of CFS is well defined and is related to both physical and mental stress.

a. true
b. false

19-2. The diagnosis of CFS can be made through

a. abnormal laboratory test results
b. assessment of the psychological state of the patient
c. exclusion of other disease
d. complaints of family and friends

19-3. Physician effort in determining the pathophysiology of CFS must exclude what?

a. psychiatric disorder
b. fundamental immune disorders
c. conditions such as HIV infection or lupus
d. all of the above

19-4. Anecdotal evidence has suggested that yoga is a useful ameliorative treatment for CFS.

a. true
b. false

19-5. Some practitioners believe CFS is a predominantly psychiatric disorder that has pronounced physiological consequences. The authors suggest this may not be a sufficient explanation. Why?

a. case definitions for CFS have been redefined several times
b. there is sufficient evidence of an organic cause
c. epidemiologic studies on CFS show no significantly higher rates of depression in CFS patients than in comparable healthy normal persons

19-6. What restricts a patient's access to CFS information?

a. low awareness of the illness among professionals
b. limited information on the disorder
c. a belief by many professionals that the disorder does not exist
d. none of the above
e. all of the above

CHAPTER 20
Integrative Approach to Endocrinology

20-1. Which of the following has been associated with insulin resistance in animal models?

a. normal levels of calcium
b. low levels of magnesium
c. low levels of molybdenum
d. high levels of magnesium

20-2. Which of the following has been shown to have a stronger association with diabetes risk?

a. soluble fiber
b. insoluble fiber

20-3. Which of the following is purported to enhance the absorption of chromium?

a. picolinate
b. chloride

20-4. World ethnobotanical data indicate that diabetes was virtually unknown in ancient times, and that there were few herbs used around the world for its treatment.

a. true
b. false

20-5. Which of the following is the correct plant part used in studies of fenugreek for diabetes?

a. root
b. leaf
c. seed
d. flower

20-6. Which of the following statements are true regarding fenugreek? (More than one answer may be correct.)

a. fenugreek has hypoglycemic activity
b. fenugreek has lipid-lowering activity
c. fenugreek can be toxic at doses greater than 2 g/d
d. fenugreek has antioxidant activity

20-7. *Gymnema*

a. has been used for the treatment of diabetes for more than 2000 years
b. has not been shown to have hypoglycemic activity in any human trials
c. has been shown to have hypoglycemic activity in animal studies

20-8. Which of the following is true about stevia? (More than one answer may be correct.)

a. stevia has been banned in the United States due to toxicity
b. stevia is an approved food additive in the United States
c. stevia is widely used as a sweetening agent in Japan
d. Alaskan natives traditionally used stevia as a diabetes treatment

20-9. Capsaicin creams have been found to be beneficial for relieving the pain of diabetic neuropathy in clinical trials.

a. true
b. false

20-10. The constituents in bilberry that act as potent antioxidants are

a. saponins
b. anthraquinones
c. anthocyanosides
d. mucilages

20-11. Excessive consumption of iodine can lead to a reversible type of hypothyroidism.

a. true
b. false

20-12. Kelp is a rich source of iodine.

a. true
b. false

20-13. The German Commission E failed to recognize bugleweed for the treatment of mild hyperthyroid conditions.

a. true
b. false

20-14. Which of the following herbs has been shown by in vitro or animal data to interfere with binding of Graves-IgG antibody to the TSH receptor at the thyroid gland? (More than one answer may be correct.)

a. motherwort
b. gromwell
c. bugleweed
d. lemon balm

20-15. The botanical name for motherwort is

a. *Lycopus virginicus*
b. *Melissa officinalis*
c. *Leonurus cardiaca*
d. *Gymnema sylvestre*

20-16. Preliminary evidence suggests that ginseng has hypoglycemic activity.

a. true
b. false

20-17. Evening primrose oil is a rich source of DHEA.

a. true
b. false

20-18. Capsaicin depletes which of the following with repeated administration?

a. serotonin
b. dopamine
c. substance P
d. epinephrine

20-19. Bugleweed appears to be safe for use during pregnancy.

a. true
b. false

20-20. The dose generally recommended per day for selenium is

a. 2000 mg
b. 200 mg
c. 20 mg
d. 200 μg

CHAPTER 21

Integrative Approach to the Gastrointestinal System

21-1. What proportion of the body's lympho-cytes resides in the GI tract?

a. 11%

b. 32%

c. 68%

d. 89%

21-2. The ratio between the number of bacte-ria residing in the adult human GI tract and the number of mammalian cells in the human body is

a. 1:1

b. 1:3

c. 2:1

d. incalculable

21-3. Deoxycholic acid has the following effects

a. protects against colon cancer

b. increases cholesterol saturation of bile

c. lowers serum cholesterol level

d. promotes hepatic encephalopathy

21-4. Antigenic cross-reactivity between *Klebsiella* and HLA-B27 may contribute to the pathogenesis of

a. rheumatoid arthritis

b. ankylosing spondylitis

c. Crohn's colitis

d. ulcerative colitis

21-5. Small bowel bacterial overgrowth may cause

a. destruction of pancreatic enzymes

b. destruction of brush border enzymes

c. both of the above

d. neither of the above

21-6. Bacterial growth in the ileum is increased by which dietary factor

a. fructose

b. protein

c. calcium

d. starch

21-7. Intraepithelial lymphocytes of the small intestine

a. are found in Peyer's patches
b. are important for oral tolerance
c. produce the antibodies that cause food allergy
d. none of the above

21-8. Increased susceptibility to yeast infection is associated with deficiency of which of the following

a. zinc
b. iron
c. vitamin A
d. all of the above

21-9. The antimicrobial properties of garlic

a. have been shown to prevent pseudomembranous colitis due to *C. difficile* toxin A
b. are greatly diminished by heating for 20 minutes
c. withstand boiling
d. are mostly found in the capsule around the cloves

21-10. Nutritional deficiency of which of the following increases transcellular absorption by active transport

a. calcium
b. magnesium
c. vitamin B_3
d. vitamin E

21-11. Normal intestinal permeability is in part maintained by the presence of

a. prostaglandin E_2
b. lactobacilli
c. secretory IgA
d. all of the above

21-12. The immune response underlying Crohn's disease is driven by

a. Th1 lymphocytes
b. atypical Th2 lymphocytes
c. IgG4 antibodies against food antigens or yeasts
d. all of the above

21-13. The immune response underlying ulcerative colitis is driven by

a. Th1 lymphocytes
b. Atypical Th2 lymphocytes
c. IgG4 antibodies against food antigens or yeasts
d. all of the above

21-14. The psychosocial intervention with the greatest evidence for benefit among patients with irritable bowel syndrome is

a. hypnotherapy
b. individualized self-management training
c. support groups
d. cognitive behavior therapy

21-15. Which of the following is true of the East Anglican Multicentre Controlled Trial of diet and Crohn's disease?

a. an individualized food exclusion diet was more effective than steroids at maintaining remission
b. symptomatic remission achieved by diet was not associated with improvement in laboratory markers of disease activity
c. dietary compliance was only 10% after the first year
d. none of the above

21-16.   Which of the following is true concerning irritable bowel syndrome?

a. pathogenic bacteria are frequently found in stool
b. there is good correlation between the results of food allergy testing and the response to diet
c. the condition is defined by the lack of any identifiable pathology, marking it as purely functional
d. no existing theory adequately describes the disparate findings of different investigators, suggesting that irritable bowel syndrome is not a single syndrome

21-17. Biofeedback has shown the most consistent benefit for which of the following conditions?

a. chronic diarrhea
b. continuous abdominal pain
c. fecal incontinence
d. esophageal reflux

21-18.   If a patient with chronic abdominal pain or distension, flatulence, and/or constipation becomes worse on a high-fiber diet, which of the following should be considered?

a. an allergic reaction to the source of increased fiber
b. excessive fermentation of fiber by intestinal microbes
c. both of the above
d. neither of the above

21-19. The most common factor producing gastroesophageal reflux appears to be

a. excess gastric acidity
b. hiatal hernia
c. relaxation of the lower esophageal sphincter caused by gastric distension
d. *Helicobacter pylori* infection

21-20.   Which of the following has been shown to increase the risk of aspirin- or NSAID-induced gastritis?

a. spicy food
b. gastric colonization with *Helicobacter pylori*
c. the use of proton pump inhibitors
d. none of the above

CHAPTER 22
Integrative Approach to Neurology

22-1. Which of the following statements about Alzheimer's disease is not true?

a. approximately 50% of the population over age 85 is believed to be affected by Alzheimer's disease

b. beta-amyloid is toxic to neurons and may be the primary cause of neuronal degeneration

c. oxidative stress is involved in the pathogenesis of Alzheimer's disease

d. Alzheimer's is associated with decreased levels of dopamine in the hippocampus

22-2. Epidemiologic studies have identified several factors involved in Alzheimer's disease except for the following:

a. increasing age

b. higher intake of total fat and cholesterol

c. an inverse relationship between Alzheimer's and COX-2 inhibitors

d. a lower incidence in women who use hormone replacement therapy

22-3. Primary symptoms of Alzheimer's disease include all of the following except

a. balance disturbances

b. short-term memory loss

c. emotional symptoms including anxiety and/or paranoia

d. speech disturbances

22-4. All of the following are true in regard to the diagnosis of Alzheimer's disease except

a. diagnosis is made on clinical grounds

b. the differential diagnosis of Alzheimer's disease may include hypocalcemia

c. magnetic resonance imaging and magnetic resonance spectroscopy may support a diagnosis of Alzheimer's disease

d. APO E4 allele may suggest a heightened risk for Alzheimer's

22-5. Which of the following is the conventional treatment approach to Alzheimer's disease?

a. anticholinergics

b. dopamine agonists

c. selective serotonin reuptake inhibitors

d. acetylcholinesterase inhibitors

22-6. Which of the following findings most supports the theory that oxidative insults are involved in the pathogenesis of Alzheimer's disease?

a. elevated levels of polyunsaturated fatty acids are found in brains of Alzheimer's patients
b. increased levels of 4-hydroxynonenal found in brains of Alzheimer's patients
c. oxidative stress products are found in senile plaques
d. reduced levels of glutathione peroxidase are found in brains of Alzheimer's patients

22-7. *Ginkgo biloba* unequivocally improves symptoms of Alzheimer's disease.

a. true
b. false

22-8. Which of the following statements about the relationship of folic acid to Alzheimer's disease is not true?

a. there is an increased concentration of homocysteine in patients with Alzheimer's disease
b. folic acid may help in increasing declining acetylcholine levels in Alzheimer's disease
c. folic acid may exert beneficial effects on cognition by improving cerebral endothelial function
d. folic acid may act as an antioxidant by reducing endothelial superoxide

22-9. Which of the following statements about the relationship of estrogen to Alzheimer's disease is not true?

a. estrogen is a growth factor
b. estrogen promotes the synthesis of acetylcholine
c. there is a higher incidence of Alzheimer's disease in premenopausal women with estrogen failure as opposed to postmenopausal women
d. preliminary studies support that estrogen may improve verbal memory and visual memory scales

22-10. Which is the proposed mechanism of how phosphatidylserine may improve symptoms of Alzheimer's disease?

a. improves membrane fluidity and enhances synaptic transduction
b. raises brain acetylcholine levels
c. raises brain catecholamine levels
d. reduces oxidative stress

22-11. Which of the following statements about acetyl-carnitine in Alzheimer's disease is not true?

a. acetyl-carnitine is structurally similar to acetylcholine
b. acetyl-carnitine raises markers of mitochondrial metabolism in the brain
c. acetyl-carnitine improves glutaminergic neurotransmission in the brain
d. acetyl-carnitine increases the production of essential neurotrophic factors

22-12. Which of the following observations supports a role for lipid lowering strategies in Alzheimer's disease?

a. elevated cholesterol may lower acetylcholine production
b. saturated fat increases the production of amyloid from amyloid precursor protein
c. high fat intake is inversely related to the risk of Alzheimer's disease
d. statins may reduce proinflammatory cytokines which are implicated in the pathogenesis of Alzheimer's disease

22-13. Which of the following statements about huperzine, a natural acetylcholinesterase inhibitor, is true?

a. huperzine has a longer half life than donepezil
b. huperzine is currently FDA approved for treatment of Alzheimer's disease
c. huperzine possesses no additional effects other than being an acetylcholinesterase inhibitor
d. huperzine is used is China as a mood enhancer

22-14. Which neurotransmitter is principally diminished in Parkinson's disease?

a. serotonin
b. dopamine
c. acetylcholine
d. histamine

22-15. The exact cause of Parkinson's disease is unknown.

a. true
b. false

22-16. Which gene has most recently been identified in familial Parkinson's disease?

a. alpha-synuclein
b. amyloid
c. nuclear factor-κβ
d. vitamin E transport gene

22-17. Which of the following findings supports the free radical hypothesis in Parkinson's disease?

a. reduced iron in peripheral cell markers
b. increased ferritin in the substantia nigra
c. reduced levels of glutathione in the substantia nigra
d. decreased cerebrospinal fluid vitamin E levels in Parkinson's disease

22-18. Which mitochondrial defect has been found in Parkinson's disease patients?

a. Na/K ATPase activity
b. complex one activity
c. cytochrome C activity
d. fatty acid oxidation shuttle pathway

22-19. Approximately how many new cases of Parkinson's disease are diagnosed each year?

a. 50,000
b. 200,000
c. 1,000,000
d. 10,000

22-20. Which of the following is not a clinical feature of Parkinson's disease?

a. akinesia
b. postural instability
c. dementia
d. hyperreflexia

22-21. Which of the following is not included in the differential diagnosis of Parkinson's disease?

a. supranuclear palsy
b. neuroleptic exposure
c. multiple cerebral insults
d. multiple sclerosis

22-22. Which of the following statements concerning conventional treatment for Parkinson's disease is not true?

a. levodopa is the most common treatment for Parkinson's disease
b. levodopa is seldom effective in monotherapy for the treatment of Parkinson's disease
c. prolonged treatment with levodopa may lead to motor complications
d. levodopa may accelerate free radical injury in dopamine-manufacturing neurons

22-23. Which of the following statements makes dopamine agonists a preferred drug of choice for first-line therapy in Parkinson's disease?

a. they are more effective in reducing symptoms than levodopa
b. they are devoid of any significant side effects
c. they are easy to tolerate in patients with comorbid dementia
d. they may exhibit neuroprotective effects

22-24. Which of the following statements concerning the use of antioxidants in Parkinson's disease is untrue?

a. antioxidants may not cross the blood–brain barrier adequately to exert physiologic effects in the central nervous system

b. antioxidants can be converted to pro-oxidants in diseased tissue

c. an ideal antioxidant would induce glutathione in the central nervous system

d. high-dose antioxidants may mask some of the symptoms of Parkinson's disease

22-25. Which of the following statements about lipoic acid is false?

a. lipoic acid is a potential metal chelator

b. lipoic acid stimulates glutathione transferase activity

c. lipoic acid may increase brain mitochondrial activity

d. lipoic acid has demonstrated moderate efficacy in Parkinson's disease management

22-26. Glutathione is readily bioavailable via the oral route.

a. true

b. false

22-27. NADH has been found to be therapeutically effective in multicenter trials of Parkinson's disease.

a. true

b. false

22-28. There is more of a predilection for multiple sclerosis in lower latitudes than in higher latitudes.

a. true

b. false

22-29. Which virus is the leading candidate in the pathogenesis of multiple sclerosis?

a. HTLV-3

b. RSV

c. HHV-6

d. HIV

22-30. Which of the following genes has been associated with an increased likelihood of multiple sclerosis in either acute or chronic lesions?

a. MAP kinase

b. APO E4

c. alpha-synuclein

d. homocysteine

22-31. Which of the following aberrations in cytokine production is most characteristic in multiple sclerosis?

a. increased IL-10 and decreased IL-12

b. decreased IL-10 and increased IL-12

c. increased IL-6

d. increased IL-1 and increased IL-6

22-32. Which of the following is not part of the differential diagnosis of multiple sclerosis?

a. subcortical ischemic disease

b. lupus

c. B_{12} deficiency

d. Shy–Drager syndrome

22-33. All of the following are FDA-approved medications for multiple sclerosis except

a. betaseron

b. avonex

c. copaxone

d. ribavirin

22-34. Which of the following are among the proposed mechanisms for the way in which interferons work?

a. enhanced production of neutralizing antibodies

b. increased production of IL-10

c. production of mild granulocytopenia

d. inhibition of histamine receptors

22-35. What percentage of patients with multiple sclerosis use alternative therapies?

a. 10%
b. 30%
c. 60%
d. 80%

22-36. All of the following observations concerning the relationship of vitamin D to multiple sclerosis are true except

a. there is a higher incidence of multiple sclerosis in the Northern Hemisphere, where vitamin D exposure is reduced
b. vitamin D increases IL-10
c. vitamin D receptive gene polymorphisms have been detected in multiple sclerosis patients
d. vitamin D therapy has lowered the incidence of relapse in multiple sclerosis patients

22-37. Omega-3 fatty acids have been definitively established as an effective therapy to prevent relapse in multiple sclerosis.

a. true
b. false

22-38. Electromagnetic therapy has demonstrated benefit in multiple sclerosis patients in regard to spasticity pain and bladder control

a. true
b. false

CHAPTER 23
Integrative Approach to Oncology

23-1. The majority of cancer patients prefer

a. chemotherapy, radiation, and/or surgery only
b. acupuncture and herbs only
c. an integrative approach
d. hospice

23-2. Clinical trials have convincingly supported the benefit of supplementing with the following vitamin, nutrient, or micronutrient to prevent certain cancers

a. beta-carotene
b. vitamin C
c. selenium
d. molybdenum

23-3. The only randomized prospective trial looking at cancer risk and selenium supplementation showed

a. a reduction in breast cancer occurrence
b. no change in skin cancer recurrence
c. a reduction in lung, colorectal, and prostate cancers
d. a reduction in lung cancer deaths

23-4. The Gonzalez regimen is not

a. related to Kelly and Gerson's programs for cancer
b. a dietary program
c. undergoing clinical trial testing for pancreas cancer
d. proven useful for cancer management

23-5. The range of complementary and alternative medicine (CAM) modalities in oncology does not include

a. botanicals
b. mind–body approaches
c. diet
d. antiprotozoan therapy

23-6. Known traditional and folk use of herbs in cancer treatment includes

a. the South American herb *Uncaria tomentosa* (cat's claw)
b. the Chinese herb *Scutellaria baicalensis*
c. the Indian herb *Phyllanthus amarus*
d. the North American herb *Ulmus rubra* (slippery elm)

23-7.   Example of foreign drugs for cancer not yet available by prescription in the United States include:

a. clodronate
b. lentinan
c. krestin (PSK)
d. all of the above

23-8.   An example of an off-label drug potentially useful as an adjunct in cancer therapy is

a. ciprofloxacin
b. Tagamet
c. doxycycline
d. all of the above

23-9.   Shark's cartilage

a. has metalloproteinase inhibitory activity
b. has antiangiogenic activity
c. is in clinical trials for cancer
d. all of the above

23-10.   Dietary programs for cancer includes all of following except

a. Macrobiotics
b. Gerson's
c. Kelly's
d. Suzuki's

23-11.   Antioxidants reduce the effectiveness of chemotherapy.

a. statement is categorically true
b. statement is categorically false
c. only in combination with hyperthermia
d. none of the above

23-12.   Which of the following chemotherapy drug(s) is/are derived from botanicals?

a. cisplatin
b. taxol
c. doxorubicin
d. camptothecin

23-13.   Well-known but unsubstantiated cancer treatments include

a. Cancell
b. Hoxsey's
c. Burton's
d. 714-X

23-14.   Hot flashes in estrogen-positive cancer patients can be treated with

a. progesterone
b. diethylstilbestrol
c. dihydroandrostenediol
d. gabapentin

23-15.   A cancer patient seeking alternative treatments

a. should be discouraged because of lack of supporting data for most regimens
b. should be warned to discontinue because it could endanger his or her life
c. should be encouraged to discuss this with his conventional physician
d. should be encouraged to avoid chemotherapy and radiation

23-16.   Melatonin (two answers)

a. has been found to have in vitro anticancer activity
b. is a hormone that controls ovulation
c. is a thalamic peptide
d. is a European health food
e. can reduce chemotherapy side effects

23-17.   The following supplement is shown by clinical trials to reduce chemotherapy side effects

a. conjugated linolenic acid
b. L-glutamine
c. beta-carotene
d. S-adenosyl methionine

23-18. Smoking marijuana as a treatment for chemotherapy-induced nausea

a. is anecdotal and unproven
b. can be prescribed as a controlled prescription
c. cannot be discussed with patients according to federal law
d. none of the above

23-19. Copper

a. is found in certain foods
b. causes angiogenesis
c. reduction could be a treatment for cancer
d. all of the above

23-20. Nausea secondary to chemotherapy may be treated with

a. emu oil
b. noni juice
c. coral calcium
d. ginger

CHAPTER 24
Integrative Approach to Osteoporosis

24-1. Osteoporosis is

a. a disease limited to bone density

b. an insignificant condition not influencing morbidity or mortality

c. a manifestation of an integrated disorder, involving metabolism in conjunction with bone and lifestyle influences

d. a soft tissue disorder causing hypocalcemia

24-2. The treatment of osteoporosis is multisystemic, involving the digestive system, endocrine system, mind, and spirit.

a. true

b. false

24-3. Bone remodeling occurs until age 55 years, when it tapers and ceases.

a. true

b. false

24-4. Osteoblasts

a. arise from monocytes

b. have no role in endocrine function

c. line the surface of bones and function in bone breakdown

d. are influenced by both local and systemic factors

24-5. Cortical bone is lost more rapidly than trabecular bone in osteoporosis.

a. true

b. false

24-6. Which of the following is incorrect?

a. osteoporosis can only occur in people over age 50 years

b. osteoporosis results from failure to reach peak bone density by age 30 years

c. osteoporosis results from bone resorption exceeding bone formation

d. osteoporosis is influenced by the body's demands on bone function

24-7. Bone loss can be influenced by estrogen or testosterone deficiency.

a. true

b. false

24-8. About 25% of patients who experience a pathologic hip fracture secondary to osteoporosis will die within 1 year of that fracture.

a. true
b. false

24-9. Osteoporosis

a. is more likely to precipitate a hip fracture in men younger than age 55 years than in women of the same age group
b. is seen only in females
c. usually begins earlier in men than in women
d. risk can be minimized

24-10. All of the following will directly test bone metabolism except

a. 24-hour urine calcium
b. plasma tartrate–resistant acid phosphatase
c. bone-specific serum alkaline phosphatase
d. urine magnesium

24-11. The generalized adaptation syndrome is an example of insufficient raw materials to meet the body's nutritional demands.

a. true
b. false

24-12. The most abundant mineral in the body is

a. Mg
b. Na
c. Ca
d. K

24-13. You are treating a 68-year-old female with osteoporosis. She has been taking calcium, vitamin D, and magnesium. In your work-up, you notice her osteocalcin level is low. Which recommendation would you make?

a. increase sun exposure
b. consider adding vitamin K 100 μg per day
c. consider administering parathyroid hormone
d. make no changes; everything that can be done is already being done

24-14. Boron will increase bowel absorption and decrease urinary excretion of calcium.

a. true
b. false

24-15. Ingestion of 1 ounce of animal protein results in the loss of ____ mg of calcium from the bones

a. 10
b. 25
c. 50
d. 100

24-16. One cup of brewed coffee causes the loss of ____ mg of calcium from bone

a. 40
b. 20
c. 10
d. 5

24-17. Fifteen billion dollars a year is spent on the treatment of osteoporosis.

a. true
b. false

24-18. In the United States in the year 2003, it is predicted that 1 million people will have pathologic hip or vertebral fractures secondary to osteoporosis.

a. true
b. false

24-19. Activities like qigong and yoga have no benefit in treating osteopenia/osteoporosis.

a. true
b. false

24-20. Stress reduction, both mental and physical, plays a major role in the treatment of osteoporosis.

a. true
b. false

CHAPTER 25
Integrative Approach to Otolaryngology

25-1. What percentage of sinusitis patients seek treatment from a primary care physician prior to being seen by a specialist?

a. 55%
b. 78%
c. 92%
d. 100%

25-2. Acupuncture is the most commonly used type of alternative medicine in patients with asthma and/or sinusitis.

a. true
b. false

25-3. The following illnesses all prompt urgent referral to an otolaryngologist except

a. facial nerve paralysis secondary to otitis media
b. unilateral otitis media in an adult
c. unilateral otitis media in a child
d. sudden-onset sensorineural hearing loss

25-4. Laryngeal papillomatosis in childhood always presents with stridor.

a. true
b. false

25-5. Echinacea has been found to have antibacterial, antiinflammatory and antiviral properties.

a. true
b. false

25-6. Tolerance to echinacea has been shown within 8 weeks of continuous use.

a. true
b. false

25-7. Clinical trials of goldenseal have been done using _____ isolated from other sources

a. hydrastine
b. canadine
c. berberine

25-8. *Astragalus* is thought to

a. enhance symptom control when combined with interferon to treat upper respiratory infections
b. increase IgE, IgM, and IgA in human nasal secretions
c. draw its therapeutic effect from numerous polysaccharides and flavonoids
d. stimulate production of interferon, T and B cells, and macrophages
e. all of the above

25-9. Bromelain is an antiinflammatory agent that has been proposed for use in the treatment of sinusitis.

a. true
b. false

25-10. Up to ___ of chronic otitis media will resolve within 3 months

a. 10%
b. 20%
c. 60%
d. 90%

25-11. Allopathic treatment of otitis media includes

a. observation
b. antibiotics
c. steroids
d. surgery
e. all of the above

25-12. Homeopathic preparations for otitis media commonly work within 72 hours of onset of therapy.

a. true
b. false

25-13. Cranial osteopathy is not recommended in children less than 2 years old.

a. true
b. false

25-14. Intranasal chiropractic techniques have been proposed to treat sinusitis.

a. true
b. false

25-15. Fresh wintergreen is an excellent choice for children with colds and fever.

a. true
b. false

25-16. Signs of obstructive apnea in children include

a. daytime somnolence
b. enuresis
c. poor school performance
d. all of the above

25-17. Dietary advice and hypnotherapy were found to be more effective than dietary advice and stress reduction in patients attempting to achieve weight loss.

a. true
b. false

25-18. Tinnitus is an uncommon clinical complaint.

a. true
b. false

25-19. Patients with tinnitus should have

a. audiogram
b. neurologic evaluation
c. thyroid function testing
d. all of the above

25-20. *Ginkgo biloba* has been demonstrated to reduce volume of tinnitus in doses of 50 μg/d.

a. true
b. false

CHAPTER 26
Integrative Approach to Pain

26-1. Chronic pain affects how many Americans?

a. 6%
b. 1 in 5
c. 1 in 3
d. 40%
e. none of the above

26-2. Traditionally doctors

a. have done a good job of managing pain for most patients
b. have felt comfortable prescribing opioid class medications
c. have used complementary and alternative medicine (CAM) modalities instead of pain medications
d. were trained in acupuncture
e. have not managed pain patients well

26-3. Opioid class medications

a. usually pose a risk for addiction
b. should only be prescribed when all other medications are not working
c. rarely have side effects
d. can develop pharmacodynamic tolerance
e. should never be given to patients with a history of addictive behavior

26-4. Pain pharmacotherapy can

a. entirely relieve most people's pain
b. obviate the need for nondrug therapies
c. be entirely safe for most patients
d. be effectively managed by most primary care physicians
e. be augmented effectively by CAM therapies

26-5. CAM therapies for pain

a. may be a good idea, but have few or no research data behind them
b. can be helpful by allowing the patient to feel less helpless
c. are an adequate substitute for conventional pain medicine
d. are rarely used by most pain sufferers
e. pose significant risks to many patients

26-6. Chronic pain

a. often does not represent significant tissue derangement or disorder
b. is defined as pain lasting greater than 3 months
c. usually means that the patient has emotional illness
d. rarely leads to diminished life function
e. always requires an exhaustive medical work-up

26-7.   CAM therapies for pain

a. include cognitive and behavioral therapies
b. should not be used in children
c. rely on acupuncture primarily
d. may be the only therapies safe for a pregnant woman
e. are ineffective for those over 70 years old

26-8.   The gate control theory of pain was developed by

a. Porter and Jick
b. Clifford Woolf
c. Watson and Crick
d. Amos and Andy
e. Melzak and Wall

26-9.   A patient's sense of being stressed

a. is a separate issue from his or her experience of pain
b. is best managed with benzodiazepines
c. usually requires a psychiatric referral
d. can amplify the pain
e. is not particularly addressed by CAM therapies

26-10.   There is no evidence that massage

a. can help a migraine headache
b. has any adverse reactions
c. lasts as well as acupuncture for back pain
d. can be helpful for the pain of trauma or fibromyalgia
e. can reduce postnatal complications

26-11.   Acupuncture

a. has strong evidence for relieving back and neck pain
b. can involve applied electric currents
c. has not been studied for use in the pediatric population
d. is the same thing as herbal medicine
e. is mostly just placebo effect

26-12.   Chinese herbs

a. are not heated because this would destroy their potency
b. contain alkaloids that can have topical pain-relieving effects
c. are only used in conjunction with acupuncture
d. have not been studied for dysmenorrhea
e. can be injected subcutaneously

26-13.   Ayurvedic medicine

a. comes originally from Tibet
b. has a diagnostic system of four basic human types
c. uses herbal remedies such as frankincense
d. is mostly based on homeopathy
e. has little to offer the pain sufferer

26-14.   Homeopathic remedies

a. are usually highly diluted
b. are probably based on the placebo effect
c. have not been studied by meta-analysis
d. are clearly useless for headache
e. have been shown to relive the pain of metastatic cancer

26-15.   Chiropractic

a. is not a whole system of medicine
b. techniques are commonly taught in medical schools
c. techniques are not uniform from one practitioner to the next
d. rarely uses low-amplitude thrusts

26-16.   Chiropractic spinal manipulation

a. is the same thing as osteopathy
b. has not been evaluated by the federal government
c. carries a significant risk of paraplegia in the lower back
d. can reduce the duration of acute low back pain
e. has been shown to ameliorate chronic pelvic pain

26-17.   Herbal remedies for pain

a. have been shown to have mechanisms similar to NSAIDs
b. will increase risk of bleeding
c. act on peripheral tissue inflammatory mechanisms only
d. probably cannot help low back pain
e. are not used topically

26-18.   Palliative care

a. is now widespread in US hospitals
b. should always include a massage therapist
c. is not necessarily multidisciplinary
d. research shows strong evidence for CAM inclusion
e. should include pastoral care

26-19.   CAM therapies for pain

a. should not be endorsed until the placebo effect can be ruled out
b. may not be able to be studied in the same way as medications
c. have little or no research to support them
d. are used by a small fringe group of the population
e. are superior to conventional pain medicine

26-20.   Pain treatment

a. is less important than treating the underlying illness
b. should always begin with appropriate pharmaceuticals
c. should be managed only by a pain specialist
d. often requires a multidisciplinary team
e. is usually adequate for most pain sufferers

CHAPTER 27
Integrative Approach to Pulmonary Disorders

27-1. The current conventional treatment approach to asthma relies most heavily on which of the following classes of medication:

a. inhaled steroids
b. leukotriene antagonists
c. theophyllines
d. ora beta-agonists

27-2. Evidence from the literature to date clearly shows that omega-3 essential fatty acid supplements are beneficial as an adjunctive treatment for asthma.

a. true
b. false

27-3. The percentage weight loss which has been shown to be helpful in improvement of pulmonary function in obese patients with asthma is approximately

a. 5%
b. 15%
c. 25%

27-4. The breathing techniques such as Hale and Buteyko, which are believed by some to be helpful in asthma management, are thought to work by which of the following mechanisms?

a. increasing hypercapnia
b. increasing hyperventilation
c. slowing respiratory rate
d. decreasing hypercapnia

27-5. The literature on biofeedback treatment for asthma has shown which of the following strategies to be effective?

a. EMG feedback on thoracic musculature
b. temperature sensor feedback
c. facial muscle relaxation feedback
d. respiratory rate feedback

27-6. Studies to date have clearly shown acupuncture treatment to be effective in which of the following situations?

a. acute asthma
b. chronic asthma
c. both
d. neither

27-7.   Studies of hypnotherapy for asthma have shown some benefit in asthma treatment. However, this benefit has been demonstrated to date only in the following populations

a.   patients with a high "susceptibility" score
b.   patients who identify stress as an asthma trigger
c.   patients with a low "suggestibility" score
d.   patients with exercise-induced asthma

27-8.   Chronic obstructive pulmonary disease (COPD) is now the fourth leading cause of death in the United States.

a.   true
b.   false

27-9.   Which of the following mind–body strategies has been shown in at least one study to be helpful in relieving symptoms of COPD?

a.   guided imagery
b.   biofeedback
c.   relaxation tapes
d.   music therapy
e.   transcendental meditation

27-10.   Of the two breathing techniques commonly taught in pulmonary rehab programs, which of the following is felt at this point to be most likely to be helpful?

a.   diaphragmatic breathing
b.   "pursed-lip" breathing

CHAPTER 28
Integrative Approach to Psychiatry

28-1. The following is true about geriatric team interventions for elderly depression:

a. nineteen (58%) of the intervention group recovered compared with only nine (25%) of the control group, a difference of 33%

b. after controlling for possible confounders in logistic regression analysis, patients of the geriatric team were twice as likely to recover than patients receiving medication alone

c. the odds of recovering with medication alone was only 0.3

d. a and c

e. all of the above

28-2. Data on split care versus integrative care are consistent with

a. patients receiving integrated treatment were seen more often when necessary, and used significantly fewer outpatient sessions overall compared to patients receiving split care; their treatment costs were, on average, lower than those of split treatment

b. patients receiving integrated treatment had longer periods of no sessions

c. patients receiving integrated treatment used more outpatient sessions overall

d. a and b

e. all of the above

28-3. Depression is the most common psychiatric disorder. In brief, the symptoms of depression include:

a. a persistent sad, anxious, or "empty" mood of any duration

b. sleeping too little but not sleeping too much

c. reduced appetite and weight loss, but not increased appetite or weight gain

d. loss of interest or pleasure in activities once enjoyed

e. all of the above

28-4. Regarding B vitamins:

a. depression has been related to oral contraceptive use, presumably through B_6 depletion

b. depressed patients have increased red blood cell aminotransferase activity or decreased urinary L-tryptophan on tryptophan loading

c. subjects who are not B_6 deficient still show benefit from B_6 when they are depressed

d. one-fourth of depressed patients have low folic acid levels, with treatment improving their depression

e. low serum folate and B_{12} are unrelated to refractory responses to antidepressant medication

28-5. Regarding other supplements:

a. 75% of depressed patients are magnesium deficient, with another 9% at borderline levels

b. studies of magnesium supplementation in depression have been disappointing

c. dramatic improvement in depression has been attributed to magnesium

d. melatonin helps sleep but does not treat depression

e. a and c

28-6. Regarding amino acid supplementation:

a. it has been reported to be helpful in some patients with depression

b. depressed patients who fail antidepressant drug treatment also fail treatment with tryptophan

c. tryptophan is not effective for depression

d. tryptophan is effective but less so than amitriptyline

e. tryptophan is as effective as amitriptyline, but combining the two gives no added benefit

28-7. Regarding omega-3 fatty acids:

a. they are effective used alone as a treatment for depression

b. phospholipids make up 60% of the dry weight of the brain and are essential for neuronal and especially for synaptic structure, playing key roles in the signal transduction responses to dopamine, serotonin, glutamate, and acetylcholine

c. the unsaturated fatty acid components of phospholipids are abnormal in depression, with excesses of eicosapentaenoic acid and other omega-3 fatty acids, and deficits of the omega-6 fatty acid arachidonic acid

d. correction of this abnormality by treatment with eicosapentaenoic acid improves depression, and these abnormalities can be explained by diet

e. all of the above

28-8. Kava kava

a. has recently been used to treat anxiety in doses of 90 mg every 3 hours

b. has no negative effects, with possibly positive effects on reaction time and cognitive processing

c. decreases anxiety without loss of mental acuity

d. is not superior to placebo

e. does not exacerbate Parkinsonism, so is especially useful for those with the disease

28-9. Therapeutic touch

a. therapeutic touch (TT) is a form of energy healing in which the practitioner's hands are moved through the patient's bioenergy field about 9 inches away from the body

b. one of the first studies and a good representation of the literature gave 90 hospitalized cardiovascular patients therapeutic touch, casual touch, or no touch, and showed that a significant decrease in state anxiety scores on the Spielberger Self-Evaluation Questionnaire occurred in the TT group compared to pretreatment ($P < .01$)

c. TT was no better in reducing state anxiety scores compared to the other 2 groups ($P <.01$)

d. in a randomized trial of therapeutic touch, 60 male and female subjects ages 36–81 hospitalized in a CCU unit were randomly assigned to receive therapeutic touch or a control noncontact group; postintervention anxiety scores were no different in the TT group compared to controls

e. a and b

28-10. Acupuncture

a. true acupuncture shows a significantly larger clinical improvement in anxiety ratings when compared to a placebo group

b. five acupuncture sessions were necessary to see a response

c. acupuncture is not effective for the treatment of anxiety

d. a and b

28-11. Regarding the etiology of schizophrenia

a. most research attention has focused on the serotonin receptor, though other theories abound

b. membrane phospholipid metabolic abnormalities have been proposed as the biochemical basis for the neurodevelopmental hypothesis of schizophrenia

c. there is substantial evidence of phospholipid and saturated fatty acid metabolic abnormalities in schizophrenia

d. patients with schizophrenia often have low levels of polyunsaturated fatty acids (PUFAs) in their red blood cells and in the brain

e. b and d

28-12. Regarding dietary therapies in schizophrenia:

a. a genetic disposition may exist which interacts with an overload of dietary fatty acids to produce symptoms

b. evidence to support the role of glutein- and casein-free diets in the treatment of schizophrenia emerged as early as 1973

c. meat-free groups are discharged earlier than patients on an unrestricted diet

d. patients improved during the meat-free period and relapsed when the meat was reintroduced

e. c and d

28-13. Regarding B vitamins and their role in schizophrenia:

a. folic acid has not been shown to be helpful among schizophrenics

b. hospitalized patients with schizophrenia had high or high-borderline RBC folate levels

c. methylfolate 15 mg/d for 6 months in addition to psychotropic medications created statistically significant gains in social and clinical recovery at 6 months

d. 50% of psychiatric patients are deficient in folic acid

e. c and d

28-14. Regarding thiamine and acetazolamide among schizophrenics:

a. diamox and thiamine interact together to reduce pyruvate dehydrogenase activity

b. patients show marked clinical improvement, with disappearance of hallucinations and decreased delusional thought and behavior

c. patients continued to do well following cessation of treatment

d. a and c

e. all of the above

28-15. Regarding omega-3 fatty acids in schizophrenia

a. Both tardive dyskinesia and the pathological symptoms of schizophrenia improved with omega-3 fatty acids

b. 10 g of Max-EPA (eicosapentaenoic acid) daily for 6 weeks resulted in significant improvement in tardive dyskinesia and psychopathological symptoms

c. RBC membrane levels of omega-3 fatty acids did not change

d. improvement on docosahexaenoic acid (DHA) was statistically significantly superior to EPA or placebo according to changes in symptom score on the Positive and Negative Syndrome Scale (PANSS)

e. a and b

28-16.   Regarding combined vitamin therapy in schizophrenia:

a. five months of multivitamin treatment showed marked differences in serum levels of vitamins, but no consistent self-reported symptomatic or behavioral differences between groups

b. the vitamins were unhelpful, the doses were too small, or other factors intervened to vitiate potential therapeutic effects

c. differences were seen in negative symptoms but not positive symptoms

d. a and b

28-17.   Regarding electroacupuncture in schizophrenia:

a. a combination of electroacupuncture and Chinese herbs was found to provide two-fold greater effectiveness with schizophrenic patients when compared to either treatment alone or to a neuroleptic alone

b. acupuncture alone, herbs alone, and neuroleptics alone were equivalent

c. chlorpromazine versus chlorpromazine + acupuncture were equivalent long-term, with marked effects appearing earlier with combined therapy than with chlorpromazine alone

d. less chlorpromazine was needed in the combined therapy group, which also displayed fewer side effects

e. all of the above

CHAPTER 29
Integrative Approach to Rheumatology

29-1. After an intravenous course of colchicine, when can one give additional colchicine?

a. the next day
b. after a minimum of 3 days
c. after a minimum of 7 days
d. after a minimum of 14 days

29-2. Which are indications for starting a uric acid–lowering agent such as allopurinol?

a. tophaceous gout
b. renal disease secondary to uric acid deposition
c. repeated attacks of gout despite prophylaxis
d. any of the above

29-3. When should you start allopurinol in a patient with an acute gouty attack and tophaceous gout?

a. immediately
b. after symptoms are resolved for about 7 days
c. after symptoms are resolved for about 2 months
d. never

29-4. Asymptomatic hyperuricemia should be treated with the following

a. steroids
b. allopurinol
c. nonsteroidal antiinflammatory medications
d. increased water intake

29-5. Which of the following may mimic or contribute to symptoms in fibromyalgia?

a. hypothyroidism
b. sleep apnea syndrome
c. hepatitis C
d. all of the above

29-6. What is the commonly reported ratio of females to males with diagnosed fibromyalgia?

a. 1:1
b. 2:1
c. 8:1
d. 16:1

29-7. All of the following have been shown to be valuable in fibromyalgia using controlled trial methods: meditation, acupuncture, aerobic exercise, S-adenosylmethionine (SAM-e), tricyclic antidepressants.

a. true
b. false

29-8. The following supplements are commonly used in fibromyalgia, despite the lack of controlled trials: calcium, magnesium, vitamin E, vitamin C, omega-3 fatty acids.

a. true
b. false

29-9. The following can be used to help increase sleep in fibromyalgia

a. tricyclic antidepressants
b. German chamomile tea
c. valarian
d. any of the above

29-10. Commonly used pharmaceuticals for fibromyalgia include: tricyclic antidepressants, SSRIs, cyclobenzaprine, and gabapentin.

a. true
b. false

29-11. Surgery can be helpful in many cases of fibromyalgia.

a. true
b. false

29-12. Soft tissue injections of tender points in fibromyalgia are usually given using

a. "dry needle"
b. saline
c. lidocaine
d. corticosteroids

29-13. Glucosamine sulfate is mainly used for the treatment of

a. rheumatoid arthritis
b. gout
c. osteoarthritis
d. diabetes

29-14. When prescribing omega-3 fatty acids

a. have the patient also decrease their intake of saturated fats and omega-6 fatty acids, which are rich sources of arachidonic acid
b. encourage more consumption of foods rich in omega-3 fatty acids like cold-water fish, flax, nuts, and green leafy vegetables
c. consider adding antioxidants such as vitamin E and selenium to reduce the pro-oxidant potential of these essential fats when they are metabolized by the body
d. remember they work in part by downregulating inflammatory mediators such as prostaglandin and leukotrienes
e. all of the above

29-15. There is excellent evidence to support the use of acupuncture for the treatment of rheumatoid arthritis.

a. true
b. false

29-16. In exploring spirituality with your patient, it is best to

a. encourage participation in a religion that you have found helpful
b. facilitate growth in helping the patient better understand what gives them meaning and purpose in their lives
c. have the answer that will heal them
d. avoid it altogether because of the risk of projecting your personal beliefs

29-17. In evaluating radiographs of someone with knee pain

a. severity of arthritis changes correlates closely with subjective symptoms
b. patients with severe arthritis with loss of joint space and severe pain should be started on glucosamine and reevaluated in 6 months
c. patients with severe arthritis with loss of joint space and severe pain should be referred for evaluation for potential knee replacement
d. arthritic changes warrant a steroid injection

29-18. In the treatment of osteoarthritis

a. glucosamine increases the shock-absorbing potential of the cartilage while chondroitin increases the viscosity of the synovial fluid

b. glucosamine increases the viscosity of the synovial fluid while chondroitin increases the shock-absorbing potential of the cartilage

c. chondroitin should be avoided in those allergic to seafood since it is derived from the chitin in crustacean shells

d. chondroitin is a small particle which is easily absorbed

29-19. All of the following statements are true regarding SAMe except

a. SAMe donates methyl groups that are involved in the synthesis of hormones, neurotransmitters, proteins, and phospholipids

b. SAMe is inexpensive

c. SAMe appears to have both structure- and symptom-modifying ability in the treatment of osteoarthritis

d. SAMe works as well as NSAIDs for pain relief without as many gastrointestinal side effects

29-20. Hypnosis for osteoarthritis pain

a. has no evidence to support any benefit.

b. only works if delivered by an experienced hypnotherapist with years of experience

c. has been found to be no better than a simple relaxation exercise in reducing pain

d. has been found to reduce arthritic pain by as much as 50%

PART IV

---

*Integrative Approaches
Through the Life Cycle*

CHAPTER 30

Integrative Approach to the Care of Children: Well-Child Care

30-1. The percentage of births taking place at home in the Netherlands is approximately

a. 5%
b. 20%
c. 35%

30-2. Neonatal mortality is equivalent in planned and unplanned out-of-hospital birth.

a. true
b. false

30-3. Children raised in the "family bed" have been shown to have a lower incidence of sleep problems and greater self-esteem later in life than children raised with separate sleeping arrangements.

a. true
b. false

30-4. Populations exposed to levels of fluoride above 4 parts per million in drinking water have been shown to have

a. increased incidence of hip fracture
b. increased incidence of osteogenic sarcoma
c. increased overall fracture incidence
d. decreased IQ

30-5. Current thinking is that a safe level of fluoridation in water supplies is

a. below 3 ppm
b. below 1 ppm
c. below 0.1 ppm

30-6. The American Academy of Pediatrics recommends drinking fluoridated water starting at age

a. 2 months
b. 6 months
c. 12 months
d. 2 years

30-7. A study of children's television programming found that a child watching television on Saturday morning is exposed to a food commercial on average every

a. 2 minutes
b. 5 minutes
c. 15 minutes

30-8. Maintaining a state of healthy immune function in a child has been shown to be effective in reducing the risk of pertussis in childhood regardless of vaccination status.

a. true
b. false

30-9. Based on the recent Danish study of autism in relation to the MMR vaccine, the risk of autism associated with MMR appears to be on the order of

a. 1 in 100,000
b. 1 in 2 million
c. no risk

30-10. Meats and dairy products are believed to account for approximately what percentage of current human exposure to PCBs and dioxins?

a. 10%
b. 50%
c. 95%

30-11. Home pesticide exposure is believed to be a risk factor for development of which of the following

a. rheumatoid arthritis
b. Parkinson's disease
c. autism
d. asthma

CHAPTER 31

Integrative Approach to Common Pediatric Conditions

31-1. Comedonal lesions without any inflammation are best treated by

a. topical retinoids
b. topical antibiotics
c. oral antibiotics
d. iso-tretinoin (Accutane)
e. washing face with soap

31-2. Comedonal lesions can be suppressed by

a. extracting them with a comedone remover
b. washing face three times a day with soap
c. changing dietary habit
d. adapalene (Diferin)
e. vitamin B_{12} supplementation

31-3. Of all the topical tretinoids, the one that has least skin irritation is

a. tretinoin 0.1%
b. tretinoin 0.05%
c. tretinoin 0.025%
d. tazarotene 0.05%
e. adapalene 0.1%

31-4. Use of iso-trentinoin is reserved for

a. patients with the pustular form of acne
b. patients with the papular form of acne
c. diabetics with acne
d. pregnant mothers with acne
e. patients with the nodulocystic form of acne

31-5. Which combination is ideal for the mild form of papulopustular acne?

a. topical erythromycin in the morning and topical clindamycin at night
b. topical tretinoin and adapalene morning and night
c. spironolactone and oral contraceptive
d. topical retinoid and systemic antibiotic
e. topical erythromycin and oral erythromycin

31-6. Which one does not act as a topical antibiotic?

a. benzoyl peroxide
b. azelaic acid
c. adapalene
d. erythromycin
e. tea tree oil

31-7. For oily skin, the vehicle for delivering medication should be

a. gel
b. cream
c. ointment
d. powder
e. water

31-8. Reduction in intake of which one of the following may improve acne?

a. protein
b. chocolate
c. carbohydrate
d. coffee
e. nuts

31-9. Which one decreases sebum production?

a. topical retinoid
b. topical antibiotic
c. topical salicylic acid
d. topical benzoyl peroxides
e. spironolactone

31-10. To which topical antibiotic is *Propionibacterium acnes* most likely to be resistant?

a. erythromycin
b. doxycycline
c. tetracycline
d. clindamycin
e. minocycline

31-11. Which alternative medicine has no antibiotic effect?

a. kampo (keigai-rengyo-to)
b. tea oil
c. sunder vati
d. azelaic acid
e. tanins

31-12. Side effects of Accutane include all except

a. dryness of skin and mucous membranes
b. increase in triglycerides
c. increase in liver enzymes
d. cardiomyopathy
e. nosebleed

31-13. Which of the following statements about vitamin A supplementation for acne is true?

a. the efficacy of vitamin A supplementation lasts far beyond the duration of treatment
b. vitamin A in high doses is relatively safe
c. hypervitaminosis A is characterized by nausea, anorexia, dry skin, and hair loss
d. vitamin A supplementation is effective even at low doses

31-14. Azelaic acid can bleach the skin.

a. true
b. false

31-15. Benzoyl peroxide can bleach clothing.

a. true
b. false

31-16. Tretinoin is listed as a category C drug.

a. true
b. false

31-17. Iso-tretinoin is listed as a category C drug.

a. true
b. false

31-18. Tazarotene does not cause photosensitivity.

a. true
b. false

31-19. Addition of clindamycin to benzoyl peroxide increases side effects.

a. true
b. false

31-20. Topical erythromycin and clindamycin are both antibacterial and antiinflammatory.

a. true
b. false

31-21. Fruit acids are helpful for acne because of their exfoliative properties.

a. true
b. false

31-22. Tea tree oil is associated with a high incidence of dryness, irritation, itching, and burning compared with benzoyl peroxide.

a. true
b. false

31-23. Azelaic acid has bacteriostatic and bactericidal properties against a variety of aerobic and anaerobic bacteria.

a. true
b. false

31-24. Vitex acts on follicle-stimulating hormone and luteinizing hormone levels to decrease progesterone levels and increase estrogen levels, and thus improve acne.

a. true
b. false

31-25. Kampo formulations are bactericidal to *Propionibacterium acnes, Staphylococcus aureus,* and *Staphylococcus epidermidis.*

a. true
b. false

31-26. Hepar sulphur in homeopathic formulation is used for painful, pus-filled acne lesions.

a. true
b. false

31-27. Sound scientific evidence exists that supports the efficacy of homeopathy for the treatment of acne.

a. true
b. false

31-28. Stress exacerbates acne.

a. true
b. false

31-29. Sound scientific evidence exists that supports the efficacy of acupuncture for the treatment of acne.

a. true
b. false

31-30. Regarding autism genetics:

a. several genes may contribute to autism, but no clear genetic linkage has been established
b. autism has clearly been established as a genetic disorder
c. while autism was once thought to affect only 1 in 500 children, recent trends indicate that its incidence is increasing, and that it may be as common as 1 in every 150 US children.
d. a and c
e. b and c

31-31. Regarding conventional therapies for autism

a. selective serotonin receptake inhibitors (SSRIs) are useful and address the underlying cause of autism, which is related to the serotonin receptor
b. autism may have many causes, all culminating in the cluster of symptoms that present as a developmental disorder
c. respiridone is quite helpful in the treatment of autism
d. donepezil is quite helpful in the treatment of autism
e. a, c, and d

31-32. Regarding magnesium:

a. its excess is involved in a number of children's developmental disorders, as well as other conditions found among developmentally disabled children (Tourette syndrome, allergy, asthma, attention deficithyperactivity disorder, obsessive–compulsive disorder, and others)

b. magnesium has been linked to multiple biochemical effects, including those on substance P, kynurenine, N-methyl-D-aspartate (NMDA) receptors, and vitamin B_6, all substances involved in the neurochemistry of autism

c. studies have reported improvement with magnesium supplementation, though usually in conjunction with vitamin B_6

d. doses of magnesium have ranged from 1–5 mg/kg of body weight per day (35–50 mg/d)

e. b and c

31-33. Regarding minerals in autism

a. the synthesis of serotonin involves calcium-requiring enzymes

b. serotonin is essential for melatonin synthesis

c. zinc levels tend to be low when levels of copper and cadmium are elevated

d. exposure to second-hand smoke and eating foods contaminated with cadmium decrease zinc levels

e. b, c, and d

31-34. Some children with fragile X syndrome (a genetic condition producing autism-like symptoms) respond to 10 mg of folic acid with B_{12} each day.

a. true

b. false

31-35. Regarding fatty acids

a. a number of disorders of neurodevelopment, including attention deficit hyperactivity disorder, dyspraxia, dyslexia, and autism have been linked to fatty acid abnormalities, including genetic defects in the enzymes involved in phospholipid metabolism, and symptom improvement has been seen following dietary supplementation with long-chain fatty acids

b. supplementation with specific fatty acids (especially omega-3 and omega-6) do not appear to have clinical utility

31-36. Regarding psychological therapies in autism, including behavior therapy

a. use of a tactile prompting device has been considered unethical

b. seeing adults imitate the behaviors of children with autism leads to increased social behavior in the children

31-37. Although atopic dermatitis has been considered mainly a disease of children, recent studies have shown that it may persist in

a. over 25% of adults

b. over 40% of adults

c. over 50% of adults

d. over 80% of adults

31-38. Which of the following statements is true concerning atopic dermatitis (AD)?

a. the lesions consist of pruritic and erythematous papules, plaques, and vesicles

b. the lesions are excoriated by scratching and often become lichenified

c. in infants, the lesions generally occur on the face, trunk, and extensor surfaces of the extremities, while from childhood on, the lesions tend to occur in the flexural areas

d. all of the above

31-39. Numerous studies have shown that **AD** is increasing in prevalence in the developing world.

a. true
b. false

31-40. Although the exact pathophysiology of AD is not known, the following are correct statements concerning this issue:

a. it has a strong genetic component and is influenced by environmental factors
b. eczematous lesions have a strong inflammatory component
c. the strong association of AD with asthma and allergic rhinitis suggest an abnormality of immune regulation
d. all of the above

31-41. The phrase "the itch that scratches" means

a. that AD is a functional illness caused by psychosomatic itching and scratching
b. that the skin lesions of AD are caused by scratching due to abnormally dry skin with a lowered threshold for itching
c. that the primary treatment for AD should be based on antipruritics such as first-generation antihistamines
d. none of the above

31-42. The following comments concerning the "hygiene hypothesis" are all true except

a. it is known that children from large families and those raised on farms have a decreased incidence of atopy
b. it is suspected that children from large families and those raised on farms have an increased incidence of viral or bacterial infection during the first year of life
c. this increased incidence of infection would presumably cause the activation of the infection-associated Th1 response rather than the Th2-associated allergic response
d. the hypothesis has been adequately tested and is now generally accepted as correct

31-43. The following types of inflammatory cells are present in eczematous lesions

a. mast cells
b. activated T cells
c. Langerhans cells
d. all of the above

31-44. There are no scientific studies indicating that the use of elimination diets can successfully treat eczema.

a. true
b. false

31-45. Which of the following statements is true?

a. stress has little role in the clinical course of AD
b. stress may have some role, but there are no physiologic mechanisms that could account for this
c. a number of studies in psychoneuroimmunology have delineated immunologic and hormonal mechanisms that help explain the role of stress in AD
d. if stress is suspected as a factor in AD, patients should immediately be referred for psychological evaluation and therapy

31-46. Mainstays of the conventional treatment approach to AD include:

a. moisturizing agents
b. avoidance of trigger factors
c. topical steroids and nonsteroidal topical immune modulators
d. antibiotics for the treatment of superinfections
e. all of the above

31-47. Triggering factors include all of the following except

a. heat, temperature changes, and any conditions that cause sweating
b. harsh soaps and detergents
c. streptococcal infections
d. psychological stress
e. aeroallergens

31-48. The use of first-generation antihistamines like diphenhydramine on a daily basis should be avoided if possible because these medications interfere with REM sleep.

a. true
b. false

31-49. The following statements are true concerning the treatment of moderate to severe AD with the higher-potency topical steroids:

a. there can be significant local side effects
b. there is some risk of systemic absorption
c. they are quite labor intensive
d. all of the above

31-50. For babies who do not breast-feed, the following statement is incorrect

a. using hydrolyzed formula makes no difference in whether these babies will develop AD
b. several studies have shown that using hydrolyzed formula had a protective effect on the incidence of food allergy and AD
c. probiotic supplementation may help to decrease the risk of AD
d. a reasonable case could be made for avoiding the most common food allergens during the first year of life

31-51. If a baby with eczema is suspected of having food allergies, the following statements are true:

a. only a double-blind placebo-controlled food challenge can be used to determine if there is food allergy
b. skin-prick testing or a radioallergosorbent test (RAST) testing should easily determine if food allergy is present
c. using a modified elimination diet with careful clinical follow-up is a reasonable clinical approach to this problem
d. food-specific IgG testing has been shown to be accurate in determining exactly what foods a baby might be allergic to

31-52. Concerning evening primrose oil, the following statements are true except

a. studies have had conflicting results as to the benefits of this treatment
b. one advantage of this treatment is that it is inexpensive and works quickly
c. evening primrose oil is safe and well tolerated in children
d. a recent study showed that interferon gamma, which was reduced in patients with AD, returned to normal with evening primrose oil treatment

31-53. Studies have shown that the following are effective topical treatments for AD

a. aloe vera
b. calendula
c. chamomile
d. licorice
e. none of the above

31-54. One randomized study found the use of cognitive therapy or autogenics to be superior to standard dermatologic education for the treatment of AD.

a. true
b. false

31-55. Concerning homeopathy, which of the following statements are incorrect?

a. skin disease represents an imbalance at an early or less severe stage

b. any successful suppressive therapy for AD would, from a homeopathic viewpoint, likely cause deeper problems at some future time

c. there have been a number of successful randomized trials concerning homeopathy and AD

d. there are case reports and patient series from the homeopathic literature claiming success in the treatment of AD

31-56. Concerning the use of traditional Chinese medicine for AD, all of the following are true except

a. there have been several controlled studies indicating that traditional Chinese herbal medicine is effective for the treatment of AD

b. although palatability has been a problem, trials of a freeze-dried capsule were also successful

c. traditional Chinese medicine generally uses a combination of a number of herbs for the treatment of AD

d. there is only poor anecdotal evidence concerning the efficacy of traditional Chinese medicine for the treatment of AD

31-57. Acupuncture has been shown to be as effective as traditional Chinese herbal medicine for the treatment of AD.

a. true
b. false

31-58. Some caution should be applied to the use of traditional Chinese medicine for AD because

a. some herbal medicines have been found to be contaminated with corticosteroids

b. there have been some reports of liver damage associated with the use of traditional Chinese medicine for AD

c. neither of the above
d. both of the above

31-59. Other alternative modalities that could be considered, but for which there is little good scientific evidence at this point include

a. craniosacral therapy
b. Reiki or healing touch
c. massage
d. hydrotherapy
e. all of the above

31-60. When instituting an elimination diet, it is important to start other modalities such as Evening Primrose Oil (EPO) or herbal medicines at the same time, so as to increase the overall chance of success.

a. true
b. false

31-61. Concerning elimination diets, the following statement is incorrect:

a. it is always important to eliminate one food at a time

b. if eliminating dairy, it is important to make sure adequate calcium is provided

c. it may take at least 1 month to know if this intervention is helpful

d. a complete multivitamin and mineral supplement is a reasonable recommendation for a child on an elimination diet

CHAPTER 32
Integrative Approach to Pregnancy

32-1. Many alternative therapies may be unsafe during pregnancy because

a. they are traditional and nonscientific
b. they are practiced by unlicensed practitioners
c. they may be used in lieu of necessary medical treatments

32-2. The most important reason for medical practitioners to understand alternative therapies that are commonly used during pregnancy is

a. to be able to provide comprehensive alternative treatment recommendations for the use of these therapies by their clients
b. to develop an open dialogue with patients in order to support their freedom of choice and provide patients with sound information on the safety and dangers of various therapies
c. to warn pregnant women never to use alternative therapies during pregnancy

32-3. Acupuncture has been shown in trials to reduce

a. incidence of shoulder dystocia
b. duration and pain of labor
c. fetal distress

32-4. The report in the *Journal of the American Medical Association* (*JAMA*) on the use of moxabustion for turning babies from breech to cephalic presentation demonstrated efficacy to be greatest when treatments were begun at

a. 28 weeks' gestation
b. 34 weeks' gestation
c. 37 weeks' gestation

32-5. Maternal stress may have a deleterious effect on fetal development, making prenatal massage a useful preventative therapy.

a. true
b. false

32-6. Women who receive massage during labor have shorter postnatal hospital stays and decreased incidence of postnatal depression.

a. true
b. false

32-7. Cardiac disorders, chronic hypertension, asthmatic mother, and convulsive disorders are excellent indications for giving prenatal massage.

a. true
b. false

32-8. That there are no case reports of adverse events from homeopathic treatments during pregnancy may be based on the fact that

a. homeopathy is unrecognized in most nations, so few studies have been conducted
b. the final products, when properly prepared, contain no detectable active chemical constituents
c. homeopathic medicines are not widely used

32-9. Homeopathic prescribing during pregnancy is based on

a. the patient's symptom picture, including physical, behavioral, and emotional symptoms
b. the safety of particularly homeopathic medication during pregnancy
c. the stage of gestation of the patient

32-10. A randomized clinical trial on the use of lavender oil for postnatal perineal comfort demonstrated

a. no benefit from the use of lavender oil
b. lower mean discomfort scores on the third and fifth days than the two control groups
c. the benefit of using undiluted oil over diluted oil

32-11. The use of comfrey during pregnancy

a. is safe as long as it is only used externally and when prescribed by a qualified professional
b. should be avoided for internal use owing to its potentially hepatotoxic effects
c. is safe when used in small doses and for short duration

32-12. Three herbs that may contain pyrrizolidine alkaloids (PAs) are

a. *Angelica sinensis, Viburnum opulus,* and *Dioscorea villosa*
b. *Matricaria recutita, Vaccinium macrocarpon,* and *Asctostaphylos uva-ursi*
c. *Symphytum officinale, Tussilago farfara,* and *Borago officinalis*

32-13. An advantage of water-based herbal preparations over hydroethanolic extracts is

a. convenience in preparation and storage
b. ease of drinking the liquid over the alcohol extract
c. decreased extraction of many of the alkaloid compounds of plants, thereby often creating a gentler medicinal preparation

32-14. An advantage of alcohol tinctures for pregnant women is that

a. they are highly concentrated and self-preserved, therefore allowing the patient to take them in small doses, and without the effort of preparation
b. they are inexpensive and paid for by insurance reimbursement
c. they are able to extract only the gentlest plant constituents, making them consistently safe

32-15. Ginger has not been proven entirely safe for use during pregnancy owing to possible inhibition of testosterone binding to its receptor site and thus theoretical interference with sexual differentiation.

a. true
b. false

32-16. Wild yam, cramp bark, and black haw are used

a. for threatened miscarriage when the primary finding is low progesterone
b. for threatened miscarriage when there is uterine cramping
c. to initiate labor when there is postdates pregnancy

CHAPTER 33

Integrative Approach to Common Conditions in Women's Health

33-1. Physiologic influences leading to premenstrual syndrome (PMS) may include

a. low luteal progesterone level
b. magnesium deficiency
c. carbohydrate intolerance
d. a, b
e. all of the above

33-2. Severe PMS is estimated to affect more than 10% of women of reproductive age.

a. true
b. false

33-3. High-fiber diets are recommended in women with PMS based on their potential effect on intestinal flora and concomitant reduction of estrogen levels.

a. true
b. false

33-4. A possible biological rationale for the effectiveness of magnesium in easing symptoms of PMS may include the following

a. promotion of muscle relaxation
b. inhibition of PGE_2
c. promotion of vascular dilatation
d. a, c
e. all of the above

33-5. Studies suggest that calcium supplementation of 1200–1600 mg/d (unless contraindicated) is a reasonable treatment option for women experiencing PMS.

a. true
b. false

33-6. Bioactive constituents of the chasteberry tree are found in the plant's root, and include essential oils, iridoid glycosides and flavonoids.

a. true
b. false

33-7. Evening primrose has been studied as a possible alternative treatment for PMS based on its abundance of linoleic and gamma-linolenic acids—two essential fatty acids that are important in the formation of the antiinflammatory prostaglandin PGE_1.

a. true
b. false

33-8. In one study, patients randomized to placebo or a standardized *Ginkgo biloba* extract (Egb761) for symptoms of PMS (congestion, breast tenderness, and altered mood) showed a statistically significant improvement in all symptoms, especially breast tenderness and fluid retention.

a. true
b. false

33-9. St. John's wort (*Hypericum perforatum*)

a. acts similarly to serotonin reuptake inhibiting preparations used for the mood symptoms of PMS and premenstrual dysphoric disorder (PMDD)
b. is often used as a botanical alternative for treating mild to moderate depressive symptoms in women with PMS
c. is contraindicated in women taking medications that increase photosensitivity or medications that are metabolized by the P450 enzyme system
d. a, c
e. all of the above

33-10. A number of other botanicals have been used clinically for the treatment of PMS. They include all of the following EXCEPT

a. kava (*Piper methysticum*)
b. andrographis (*Andrographis paniculata*)
c. dong quai root (*Angelica sinensis*)
d. wild yam (*Dioscorea villosa*)

33-11. Several large studies have demonstrated the effectiveness of cognitive behavioral therapy (CBT) in alleviating negative symptoms in women with PMS.

a. true
b. false

33-12. Light therapy has been investigated as a possible therapeutic intervention in PMS given the hypothesis that the negative mood symptoms experienced in PMDD may be due to a maladaptive response to light in the symptomatic luteal phase or to a disturbance in the circadian clock itself.

a. true
b. false

33-13. Manipulative therapies utilized in the treatment of PMS include all of the following except

a. massage
b. reflexology
c. chiropractic
d. yoga

33-14. In one small study of individualized homeopathic prescription for PMS, 90% of those receiving active treatment compared to 37.5% of those receiving placebo showed an improvement in symptoms of at least 30%.

a. true
b. false

33-15. Types of vaginitis include:

a. bacterial or nonspecific
b. trichomonal
c. hormonal
d. candidal

33-16. Lactobacilli

a. produce lactic acid and help maintain pH
b. interfere with bacterial adherence to the vaginal wall
c. can prevent overgrowth of anaerobic bacteria by producing H_2O_2
d. may have direct toxic effects against *Gardnerella*

33-17. Botanicals used in the treatment of bacterial vaginitis include:

a. garlic
b. goldenseal
c. stinging nettle
d. feverfew

33-18. True statements regarding the use of garlic in vaginitis include:

a. it can be used intravaginally and/or orally
b. it has potent antibacterial and antiviral effects
c. allicin is the most active component
d. effectiveness of garlic has been proven in the literature

33-19. Betadine is used to treat vaginitis and is safe in pregnancy.

a. true
b. false

33-20. Estrogen plays a role in the development of vaginitis

a. low levels of estrogen can lead to thin, atrophic, and inflamed vaginal tissue
b. high levels of estrogen cause inflammation
c. topical estrogens are not indicated
d. oral estrogens are not indicated

33-21. Vitamins B_2 and B_6 have been shown to act synergistically with estradiol in rat models.

a. true
b. false

33-22. Unprocessed forms of soy include:

a. tofu
b. miso
c. salted soy beans
d. brown rice

33-23. True statements regarding nonspecific and trichomonal vaginitis include:

a. six million cases of vaginitis in the United States annually are caused by *Trichomonas*
b. nonspecific vaginitis is not a reportable disease
c. trichomoniasis is a reportable disease
d. the routine use of douches helps prevent both forms of vaginitis

33-24. In vaginitis, bacterial survival is dependent on vaginal pH.

a. true
b. false

33-25. Vitamin E deficiency can depress immune responses to antigens.

a. true
b. false

33-26. Women in Italy with uterine myomas report more frequent consumption of

a. dairy products
b. red meat and ham
c. coffee
d. green vegetables

33-27. Cigarette smoking increases the risk of uterine fibroids.

a. true
b. false

33-28. Herbs traditionally used to treat the heavy bleeding associated with fibroids include:

a. nettles
b. mullein
c. shepherd's purse
d. bethroot

33-29. Reducing estrogenic influence is a principle in the integrative approach to fibroids.

a. true
b. false

33-30. A review of Esogenic Colorpuncture Therapy treatment for uterine fibroids showed

a. fibroids disappeared in less than 25% of cases
b. fibroids deceased in size in 45% of women
c. no improvement in back and abdominal pain
d. positive change in sleeping

33-31. Two uncontrolled studies of Chinese herbs show improvement in symptoms or fibroid size in approximately 90% of women with uterine fibroids.

a. true
b. false

33-32. Although not well studied, mind–body approaches in the treatment of fibroids include:

a. yoga
b. hypnosis
c. imagery focusing on releasing blocked energy
d. relaxation training

CHAPTER 34
Integrative Approach to Menopause

34-1. Of the following list of perimenopausal symptoms, which is the least common?

a. vaginal dryness
b. fatigue
c. menstrual irregularities
d. vasomotor symptoms

34-2. There is little difference in the symptom intensity between women experiencing menopause due to surgical, ablative, or natural causes.

a. true
b. false

34-3. During the 12 months that (retrospectively) determine the date of onset of the menopause, no contraceptive methods are necessary to avoid inadvertent pregnancy.

a. true
b. false

34-4. Which of the following are important for the evaluation of a perimenopausal woman?

a. assessment of her current activity level
b. assessment of her current dietary intake and habits
c. evaluation of her medical and family histories for additional risk factor analysis
d. her understanding the length of time she may need to use contraception
e. all of the above
f. none of the above

34-5. A blood follicle-stimulating hormone (FSH) level is sufficient, by itself, to assess the presence of menopause in a recently amenorrheic woman.

a. true
b. false

34-6. The perimenopause is a poor time to address life style issues and risk identification with your patient because she already has so much to deal with that it will likely adversely affect your relationship with her.

a. true
b. false

34-7.   Which of the following is true?

A. the regular performance of physical exercise is helpful for the encouragement of restful sleep as well as for the prevention and treatment of a variety of medical and psychological problems, including those associated with the perimenopause/menopause

B. walking has been proven effective for the reduction of cardiovascular disease risk in women

a. A
b. B
c. both
d. neither

34-8.   Which of the following is true?

A. alcohol and grapefruit juice ingestion may transiently increase plasma levels of bioavailable (exogenously administered) estrogen

B. blood levels of exogenously administered estrogen by oral or transdermal routes are equally affected by alcohol and grapefruit juice

C. growth hormone, androgen (including testosterone), insulin, and glucocorticoids reduce sex hormone–binding globulin levels and so increase circulating bioavailable estrogen levels as well

a. A and B
b. B and C
c. A and C

34-9.   Which of the following is true?

A. initially, when prescribing estrogen supplementation therapy for a symptomatic patient, it is best to begin with a very high dose (to be sure to stop her symptoms) and then titrate the dose down over several months

B. if the only symptom your patient is complaining of is vaginal dryness and associated dyspareunia, it is best to prescribe systemic estrogen first, as other symptoms as will inevitably start

C. if your patient is not responding to the highest single-dose forms of estrogen available, your first move should be to increase the dosage incrementally until you find the dose that controls her symptoms

D. since Premarin (conjugated equine estrogens) has been used in so many studies and has been on the market so long, there is no reason to use any of the other available formulations on the market

a. A
b. B
c. C
d. all of the above
e. none of the above

34-10. Different selective estrogen-receptor modulators (SERMs) exert selective agonist or antagonist effects on different estrogen target tissues. Which of the following is true?

A. raloxifene reduces the incidence of vertebral fracture, but does not reduce the risk of hip fracture

B. raloxifene is associated with a worsening of vasomotor symptoms and vaginal atrophy in some women

C. raloxifene affects serum lipids similarly to oral estrogen, but unlike estrogen does not increase triglycerides

D. selective receptor modulators are unlikely to evolve into major agents in the prevention and treatment of problems associated with the menopause in the future

a. A, B, and D
b. A, B, and C
c. B, C, and D
d. A only
e. B only
f. B and C

34-11. Which of the following is false regarding progestins?

A. medroxyprogesterone acetate (MPA), norethindrone, and norgestimate are all synthetic progestins available in combination hormone replacement therapy products in the United States

B. progesterone dosing must be exact because of its association with progesterone-dependent neoplasia

C. norethindrone or norgestimate *may* be associated with less breakthrough bleeding for women using the continuous, combined hormone supplementation regimen

D. topical progesterone cream application (20–40 mg/d of a 400–600 mg/ounce concentration preparation) is insufficient for endometrial protection and the prevention of bone loss, but may be quite helpful for the treatment of vasomotor symptoms

a. D
b. C
c. A
d. B

34-12. Off-label testosterone therapy in women should be closely monitored because of the seriousness of the potential adverse effects. These effects may include all but which one of the following?

a. reduction of high-density lipoprotein (HDL) cholesterol levels
b. hepatic function derangements
c. voice deepening
d. bone loss
e. acne
f. hirsutism

34-13. Which of the following is true regarding menopausal estrogen therapy and breast cancer?

A. studies have been conflicting as to whether estrogen increases the likelihood of breast cancer. If there is a slight risk increase, it remains unclear whether estrogen increases the incidence of new cancers or may stimulate the growth of a preexisting tumor
B. alcohol has been linked to an increase in risk of breast cancer, and the effect may be enhanced in association with hormone replacement therapy
C. studies have consistently shown that women with breast cancer who use (or have used) menopausal hormone supplementation are diagnosed at earlier stages, develop better differentiated tumors, and have less metastatic disease and significantly lower mortality rates than those who have not used estrogen or estrogen/progestin therapy

a. A
b. B
c. C
d. all
e. none

34-14. Limitations of the Women's Health Initiative trial include all of the following except

a. it used only oral Premarin (conjugated equine estrogens) or medroxyprogesterone acetate (a synthetic progestin in combination with Premarin marketed as PremPro) formulations applied against placebo, excluding all other formulations, so any generalizations cannot be conclusively extrapolated to those other formulations
b. it excluded women who were currently experiencing a significant number of hot flushes from the study group. This resulted in the exclusion of a large number of women in the early menopausal years
c. it was retrospective and included small numbers compared to previous studies
d. it has not helped answer the question whether postmenopausal hormone therapy initiates the development of new breast cancers or accelerates the growth of a preexisting malignant focus allowing for earlier detection and treatment
e. it will not answer whether bioidentical hormones will increase the risk of breast cancer, regardless of the mechanism involved.

34-15.   Which of the following is true regarding hormones and epithelial ovarian cancer?

a.   ovarian cancer is usually caught at an earlier stage in those on hormone replacement

b.   used together, annual transvaginal ultrasound and serum CA125 surveillance are an effective tool and have few false-positive results when used in the general, low-risk population

c.   use of oral contraceptives for 5 or more years (during the reproductive years) is an accepted risk reduction strategy, even for women with a positive family history of epithelial ovarian cancer

d.   prophylactic bilateral oophorectomy performed in high-risk women reduces, but does not eliminate, the risk of ovarian cancer, as peritoneal carcinomas may still occur

e.   ovarian cancer has not been historically linked to the use of menopausal hormone therapy, but two recent prospective cohort studies and one meta-analysis found an increased risk with 10 or more years of use

34-16.   Which of the following is false?

a.   hormone replacement therapy (HRT) reduces the risk of colorectal cancer, and this finding has been consistent across all studies to date

b.   hormone replacement therapy is generally associated with increased bone mineral density (BHD) and the clinical endpoint of reduced fracture risk of *both* the hip and spine

c.   monitoring of BMD is important in women on HRT because there exist some poor or nonresponders to estrogen's antiresorptive effect on their bones

d.   estrogen treatment has been consistently found to reverse the effects of established, severe Alzheimer's disease

e.   estrogen may be most effective for the prevention or delay of the onset of the debilitating effects associated with Alzheimer's disease when it is begun early in the menopausal period (and used for more than 10 years) when the changes are occurring in the brain that lead to the phenotypic expression of the disease

34-17.   Which of the following is true regarding hormones and glucose metabolism?

A.   oral contraceptives reduce insulin sensitivity in normal women

B.   prospective studies of postmenopausal women with type 2 diabetes have shown that estrogen supplementation improves all glucose metabolic parameters

C.   estrogen replacement, especially with natural bioidentical estrogens, may counteract the age-related changes of glucose metabolism

D.   only transdermal estrogen supplementation has been shown to exert positive effects on glucose metabolism

E.   oral bioidentical, micronized progesterone has less of a blunting effect than oral synthetic progestins on the positive effects of estrogen on glucose metabolism

a.   A only
b.   A, B, D, and E
c.   A, B, C, and E
d.   B and C
e.   D only

34-18.   Heart disease is the number one cause of death in women in the United States and exceeds the number of breast cancer deaths by 10-fold. Which of the following primary prevention measures may help avert or lessen the phenotypic expression of coronary heart disease?

A.   regular physical activity
B.   nutrition education and follow-up
C.   encouragement of social involvement (prevent isolation)
D.   smoking cessation
E.   assertive treatment of hypertension and hyperlipidemia
F.   stress reduction education

a.   all of the above
b.   A, B, D, and E
c.   all but C
d.   A, C, and F
e.   all but C and F

34-19. Which of the following statements is false?

a. the Multiple Outcomes of Raloxifene Evaluation (MORE) trial showed that raloxifene reduces the occurrence of cardiac events in all, not just high-risk, women

b. follow-up reports drawn from the 20 years of data from the Nurses Health Study revealed (in 2000) that the risk for *primary* cardiac events was lower among current, even short-term, hormone users as compared to never-users. In 2001, they reported that the risk for *recurrent* major coronary events in the same population increased among short-term users, but decreased with longer term use as compared to never-users

c. the randomized, prospective Heart and Estrogen/Progestin Replacement Study (HERS) was a *secondary prevention* trial of postmenopausal women who had not taken hormone replacement immediately before the study, who were given placebo or combination conjugated equine estrogen and medroxyprogesterone acetate. The study showed no reduction of cardiac events (as compared to the placebo group) during the 3-year period, but did show an increase in events in the treatment arm during the first year only

34-20. Which of the following regarding thyroid function is true?

A. it is important to screen women for thyroid dysfunction because there is a gender prevalence of the disease and many of the symptoms overlap with those of the perimenopause and menopause

B. untreated, subclinical thyroid dysfunction has been associated with serious circulatory and cardiovascular disease in older adults

C. oral estrogen may prompt the need for a dosage change of thyroid medication due in part to the induction of thyroid-binding globulin (TBG) synthesis by the liver. This does not occur with the use of transdermal preparations

a. A and B
b. all
c. none
d. A and C

CHAPTER 35

Integrative Approach to Geriatrics

35-1. In an examination of risk factors in a community-based elderly population, of the 423 falls deemed to be due to causes within the person, only 50% were ascribed to a single factor.

a. true
b. false

35-2. Delirium leads to falls, and the most common causes of delirium are metabolic encephalopathies and drug intoxications.

a. true
b. false

35-3. Regarding osteoporosis:

a. taking folic acid has not been shown to help
b. L-lysine was once popular but has not turned out to be effective as a preventive agent
c. strontium is helpful
d. reducing boron is helpful
e. reducing vitamin K intake can be helpful

35-4. Regarding SAM-e and osteoarthritis:

a. S-adenosylmethionine (SAM-e) had been used on 10,000 osteoarthritis patients by 1988
b. in a double-blind trial, SAMe 600 mg/day was as effective as naproxen in 676 patients with osteoarthritis of the hips and knees
c. the onset of action is slower than that of nonsteroidal antiinflammatory drugs (NSAIDs) and the benefits persist longer than NSAIDs when it is stopped
d. a and c
e. all of the above.

35-5. Regarding vitamin D and osteoarthritis

a. in a study of 516 subjects, those consuming 4000 IU/day of vitamin D were twofold less likely to have serious osteoarthritis knee disease than those consuming less than 1000 IU/day

b. 516 subjects were seen from 1983–1985 and rechecked in 1992–1993 as part of the Framingham follow-up with a relative risk for progression of osteoarthritis in the lower tertile versus the upper tertile for vitamin D intake of 4.0 ($P = .009$) and for serum vitamin D levels at baseline, 2.9 ($P = .05$)

c. in those with disease at baseline, the relative risk for loss of cartilage by comparison radiographs in the lowest tertile compared to the highest was 5 and for osteophyte growth 6

d. a and c

e. all of the above

35-6. Regarding Tai Chi

a. Tai chi, short for Tai chi chuan, is a traditional Chinese exercise developed centuries ago as a martial arts form to ward off foreign invaders

b. it has been practiced in China since then, primarily by elderly individuals, as an art form, religious ritual, relaxation technique, exercise, and form of self-defense

c. during the past century Tai Chi has been promoted in China, and more recently in the West, for the improvement and maintenance of health as well as the treatment of chronic illness

d. a and c

e. all of the above

35-7. Regarding qigong

a. Qigong has not been shown to be useful for preventing falls, although it reduces hypertension, helps respiratory disease, and reduces the side effects of cancer

b. studies suggest that practicing Qigong exercises may favorably affect many functions of the body, permit reduction of the dosage of drugs required for health maintenance, and provide greater health benefits than the use of drug therapy alone

c. for hypertensive patients, combining Qigong practice with drug therapy did not reduce the incidence of stroke and mortality, but did reduce the dosage of drugs required for blood pressure maintenance

d. a and c

e. all of the above

35-8. MacDonald's five dimensions to spirituality include:

a. cognitive orientation towards spirituality (i.e., nonreligious spiritual beliefs and the perception of spirituality as having direct relevance to personal day-to-day functioning)

b. religious attendance dimension

c. social well-being

d. conventional beliefs

e. conformity

PART V

Legal and Ethical Issues

CHAPTER 36

Legal and Ethical Issues in Integrative Medicine

36-1. Physicians can obtain some protection against malpractice actions by having patients sign an informed consent form; these forms:

a. describe the nature of the therapy to the patient, including how it is viewed by the medical community
b. the potential risks and benefits of the proposed therapy
c. show that the patient consented to the procedure with knowledge of the risks
d. all of the above

36-2. In order to practice acupuncture, a physician must

a. have completed a 200-hour postgraduate training program
b. have registered his or her practice with the board
c. there are no requirements; its part of a physician's broad scope of practice
d. it depends on the state; in some states, even physicians cannot practice acupuncture

36-3. When practicing in a multidisciplinary setting such as a group practice, a physician can insulate himself or herself from malpractice liability against the other practitioners by making sure that the complementary alternative medicine (CAM) practitioners are organized and billed as a separate legal entity.

a. true
b. false

36-4. If a CAM practitioner to which a physician referred a patient harms the patient through the CAM practitioner's negligence, the physician could be subject to discipline by the medical board if

a. no "if's"; the referring physician can be disciplined
b. the state has adopted the Federation of State Medical Boards (FSMB) guidelines about responsible referral
c. the practitioner was not properly trained and the physician should have known
d. b and c

36-5. Under FDA requirements for dietary supplements, vitamins may not be sold if

a. they make an unproved claim that the vitamin can prevent or treat a disease
b. the potency exceeds 150% of the RDA
c. they have not been preapproved by FDA for sale
d. they contain botanical products that have not been preapproved

36-6. Is it true that a physician counseling a patient must follow the federal requirement that claims be limited to "structure and function" claims and not as a benefit for a particular disease?

a. yes, because federal law overrides state law
b. no, because the FDA does not have jurisdiction over the practice of medicine
c. no, because a physician's medical training qualifies him or her to make such statement
d. b and c

36-7. Numerous manufacturers offer diagnostic devices, test kits, and various treatments based upon alternative theories about health and disease. In evaluating whether to use such devices or tests, physicians should be aware that

a. the physician may use these devices and tests whether or not the FDA approved them, as the FDA does not have jurisdiction over medical practice
b. the physician must be careful about unapproved devices, as the FDA has jurisdiction over the sale of these devices in interstate commerce and can seize unapproved devices
c. many manufacturers make exaggerated claims about these products because FDA enforcement cannot keep pace with the amount of sales activity
d. b and c

36-8. A nationally board certified rolfer (a respected form of deep tissue massage) has met all of the professional criteria in his field. Neither the State of New Alabama nor its counties license massage therapists. In New Alabama, the rolfer

a. may not practice rolfing because massage therapy is not authorized for practice there
b. may practice since he or she has met all of the national certification criteria and the state has not adopted differing requirements
c. may not practice until providing notice (registering) to the state that he will be rolfing there
d. may practice because rolfing is a specialized technique and therefore is not massage

36-9. Next door in New Georgia, its typical massage licensing statute defines massage as "the manipulation of soft tissue for the purpose of obtaining a health benefit." Alexander technique is another form of bodywork, a movement reeducation therapy that involves touching patients while instructing them in better balance and posture. In New Georgia, an Alexander practitioner would

a. have to have a massage license because the client would be touched
b. would not need a license because touching by itself is not soft tissue manipulation
c. need to get a license as a physical therapist, because movement reeducation can only be done by a PT
d. not be able to practice

36-10. For a CAM practitioner working outside their licensed scope, on-site, and under the supervision and license of a physician, which of the following is NOT necessary?

a. the physician must have first seen the patient during the course of treatment

b. the physician must continually train and assess the skill level of the practitioner

c. the physician must be physically present in the room at the time the practitioner works with the patient

d. the physician must review and sign notes for services rendered

36-11. If physicians wish to create separate practice structures, one for conventional care paid under conventional insurance/managed care contracts, and another for fee-for-service CAM arrangements, it is important to remember when entering into participation agreements with preferred provider organizations (PPOs) and health maintenance organizations (HMOs) and that

a. PPO/HMOs are likely to pay significant rates for integrative care since they recognize the value of this care

b. PPO/HMOs require special certification in integrative medicine

c. separate entities with separate tax IDs should be set up to enter these contracts to ensure that they are only binding for the conventional practice and not on the integrative/CAM entity

d. PPOs/HMOs have separate contracting arrangements for integrative/CAM practices

36-12. A common billing issue that arises when using multidisciplinary, nonstandard approaches is that

a. services delivered the same day may not each be reimbursable

b. there is not a current procedural terminology (CPT) code available for the CAM procedure

c. the ICD-9 and CPT code pairs do not match expected practice

d. all of the above

36-13. Physicians whose focus is CAM care and who find most of their services are not covered by Medicare may be well advised to opt-out of the Medicare program. A physician can opt-out in just the setting where they deliver CAM care, and continue to accept Medicare at a hospital or other conventional site.

a. true

b. false

36-14. If a physician discusses homeopathy as part of an office visit in which a range of conventional and other treatments is considered, the entire visit becomes nonreimbursable by major medical insurance polices because the visit delivered "medically unnecessary" care.

a. true

b. false

36-15. The right of patients to access the health care of their choice is anchored in

a. the right of privacy implied in the US Constitution

b. the Ninth Amendment

c. well-established principles of common law

d. no basis; no such right has been recognized

36-16. Legislation in a number of states supporting a physician's right to practice integrative medicine states that

a. physicians should be able to recommend and sell botanical and herbal products

b. medical boards cannot discipline a physician simply for using CAM approaches

c. physicians should be able to retain CAM practitioners in their centers without fear of discipline

d. physicians' use of CAM in their private practice should not affect their right to retain hospital privileges

36-17. Designing integrative practice structures that create multiple entities must take into account:

a. anti-kickback regulations
b. Stark ownership self-referral prohibitions
c. corporate practice of medicine restrictions
d. a and b

36-18. The most common difficulty integrative physicians face in using CPT codes is

a. failing to give notice to patients about clearly noncovered services
b. using incorrect modifiers
c. upcoding evaluation and management (office) visits to a higher level of service
d. not entering the amount of time spent on the office visit

36-19. Specific privileging of integrative practices in a hospital setting allows a hospital to

a. ensure that all of the medical staff are happy with who is involved with these services
b. meet new Joint Commission on Accreditation of Healthcare Organizations (JCAHO) guidelines about integrative practice
c. meet state medical board requirements for the provision of services through the medical staff
d. limit the methods practiced at the hospital to those specific therapies that fit with the hospital's guidelines, risk management strategies, and comfort of the medical staff

36-20. In *Rutherford*, the Supreme Court held that

a. there is no constitutional right to access the health care of one's choice
b. not even the patient's status as "terminal" excludes him or her from FDA restrictions on the use of unapproved drugs
c. patients may, under limited circumstances, have access to unapproved drugs
d. laetrile is a nutritional product and so could be freely used as a cancer therapy

ANSWERS

► CHAPTER 1

1.	a
2.	b
3.	a, c, d
4.	d
5.	a
6.	d
7.	a
8.	b
9.	a
10.	a

► CHAPTER 2

1.	a
2.	d
3.	d
4.	d
5.	c
6.	b
7.	a
8.	d
9.	c
10.	a

► CHAPTER 3

1.	c	**11.**	a
2.	b	**12.**	c
3.	a	**13.**	c
4.	d	**14.**	d
5.	b	**15.**	c
6.	b	**16.**	b
7.	b	**17.**	d
8.	b	**18.**	a
9.	c	**19.**	d
10.	c	**20.**	a

► CHAPTER 4

1.	b	**11.**	c
2.	d	**12.**	c
3.	b	**13.**	a
4.	d	**14.**	a
5.	c	**15.**	b
6.	b	**16.**	c
7.	a	**17.**	b
8.	d	**18.**	c
9.	c	**19.**	d
10.	d	**20.**	a

▶ **CHAPTER 5**

1. b
2. b
3. e
4. b
5. a
6. a
7. a
8. a
9. a
10. a
11. b

▶ **CHAPTER 6**

1. a
2. a
3. c
4. b
5. a
6. a
7. a
8. a
9. a
10. a

▶ **CHAPTER 7**

1. b
2. b
3. b
4. e
5. c
6. b
7. a, b
8. a, d
9. d
10. b
11. b, c
12. a, b, e
13. a, c, d, e
14. a

▶ **CHAPTER 8**

1. b
2. a
3. a
4. a
5. d
6. a
7. c
8. a
9. e
10. a
11. a
12. a
13. a
14. a
15. e
16. a
17. a
18. a
19. a
20. e

▶ CHAPTER 9

1.	b	12.	a
2.	b	13.	a
3.	a	14.	c
4.	b	15.	a
5.	a, b, c	16.	a
6.	b	17.	a
7.	c	18.	a
8.	d	19.	a
9.	a	20.	a
10.	a	21.	a
11.	d		

▶ CHAPTER 11

1.	a	12.	b
2.	d	13.	a
3.	a	14.	d
4.	a	15.	a
5.	a	16.	d
6.	a	17.	a
7.	d	18.	a
8.	a	19.	a
9.	d	20.	d
10.	a	21.	d
11.	b		

▶ CHAPTER 10

1.	a	11.	c
2.	b	12.	b
3.	d	13.	a
4.	d	14.	b
5.	d	15.	d
6.	d	16.	b
7.	a	17.	b
8.	c	18.	c
9.	b	19.	d
10.	d	20.	b

▶ CHAPTER 12

1.	b	11.	c
2.	d	12.	d
3.	c	13.	c
4.	c	14.	d
5.	c	15.	d
6.	c	16.	a
7.	a	17.	c
8.	c	18.	d
9.	b	19.	e
10.	c	20.	a

▶ CHAPTER 13

1.	a	**9.**	a
2.	a	**10.**	a
3.	a	**11.**	a
4.	b	**12.**	a
5.	b	**13.**	a
6.	a	**14.**	b
7.	b	**15.**	b
8.	a	**16.**	a

▶ CHAPTER 14

1.	b	**11.**	a
2.	d	**12.**	b
3.	d	**13.**	b
4.	b	**14.**	d
5.	c	**15.**	a
6.	c	**16.**	a
7.	d	**17.**	b
8.	a	**18.**	a
9.	a	**19.**	a
10.	b	**20.**	b

▶ CHAPTER 15

1.	b
2.	c
3.	b
4.	a
5.	c
6.	b
7.	a
8.	a
9.	a
10.	a
11.	d

▶ CHAPTER 16

1.	b
2.	a, c, d
3.	c
4.	b
5.	a, b, d
6.	c
7.	a
8.	a, b, c
9.	c
10.	c
11.	a, c, d
12.	b, c, d, f
13.	b

► CHAPTER 17

1.	b	12.	a
2.	d	13.	a, b, c
3.	b	14.	a
4.	a, b, c, d	15.	a
5.	e	16.	b
6.	b	17.	a
7.	b	18.	a
8.	a	19.	a
9.	a	20.	a
10.	a, c	21.	a
11.	a	22.	a

► CHAPTER 18

1.	b	11.	b
2.	b	12.	c
3.	b	13.	b
4.	b	14.	a
5.	d	15.	b
6.	b	16.	a
7.	d	17.	c
8.	e	18.	b
9.	b	19.	a
10.	a	20.	e

► CHAPTER 19

1.	b
2.	c
3.	d
4.	a
5.	c
6.	e

► CHAPTER 20

1.	b	11.	a
2.	b	12.	a
3.	a	13.	b
4.	b	14.	b, c, d
5.	c	15.	c
6.	a, b, d	16.	a
7.	a, c	17.	b
8.	c	18.	c
9.	a	19.	b
10.	c	20.	d

► CHAPTER 21

1.	c	11.	d
2.	a	12.	a
3.	b	13.	b
4.	b	14.	a
5.	c	15.	a
6.	d	16.	d
7.	b	17.	c
8.	d	18.	c
9.	b	19.	c
10.	a	20.	b

▶ CHAPTER 22

1.	d	20.	d
2.	c	21.	d
3.	a	22.	b
4.	b	23.	d
5.	d	24.	d
6.	a	25.	d
7.	b	26.	b
8.	b	27.	b
9.	c	28.	b
10.	a	29.	c
11.	c	30.	a
12.	d	31.	b
13.	a	32.	d
14.	b	33.	d
15.	a	34.	b
16.	a	35.	c
17.	c	36.	d
18.	b	37.	b
19.	a	38.	a

▶ CHAPTER 23

1.	c	11.	d
2.	c	12.	b, d
3.	c	13.	c
4.	b	14.	d
5.	d	15.	c
6.	c	16.	a, e
7.	d	17.	b
8.	d	18.	d
9.	d	19.	c
10.	d	20.	d

▶ CHAPTER 24

1.	c	11.	a
2.	a	12.	c
3.	b	13.	b
4.	d	14.	a
5.	b	15.	b
6.	a	16.	a
7.	a	17.	a
8.	a	18.	a
9.	a	19.	b
10.	d	20.	a

▶ CHAPTER 25

1.	b	11.	e
2.	b	12.	a
3.	c	13.	b
4.	b	14.	a
5.	a	15.	b
6.	b	16.	d
7.	c	17.	b
8.	a	18.	b
9.	a	19.	d
10.	c	20.	b

▶ CHAPTER 26

1.	b	11.	b
2.	e	12.	b
3.	d	13.	c
4.	e	14.	a
5.	b	15.	c
6.	a	16.	d
7.	d	17.	a
8.	e	18.	e
9.	d	19.	b
10.	a	20.	d

► CHAPTER 27

1. d
2. b
3. b
4. a, c
5. c
6. a
7. a
8. a
9. a, c, d
10. b

► CHAPTER 28

1. d
2. d
3. d
4. a
5. e
6. a
7. b
8. c
9. b
10. d
11. e
12. b
13. c
14. b
15. e
16. d
17. e

► CHAPTER 29

1. c
2. d
3. c
4. d
5. d
6. c
7. a
8. a
9. d
10. a
11. b
12. c
13. c
14. e
15. b
16. b
17. c
18. a
19. b
20. d

► CHAPTER 30

1. c
2. b
3. b
4. a, c, d
5. b
6. b
7. b
8. b
9. c
10. c
11. b

▶ CHAPTER 31

1.	a	32.	e
2.	d	33.	e
3.	e	34.	a
4.	e	35.	a
5.	d	36.	b
6.	c	37.	c
7.	a	38.	d
8.	c	39.	a
9.	e	40.	d
10.	a	41.	b
11.	e	42.	d
12.	d	43.	d
13.	c	44.	b
14.	a	45.	c
15.	a	46.	e
16.	a	47.	c
17.	a	48.	a
18.	a	49.	d
19.	b	50.	a
20.	a	51.	c
21.	a	52.	b
22.	b	53.	e
23.	a	54.	a
24.	b	55.	c
25.	a	56.	d
26.	a	57.	b
27.	b	58.	d
28.	a	59.	e
29.	b	60.	b
30.	d	61.	a
31.	b		

▶ CHAPTER 32

1.	c	9.	a
2.	b	10.	b
3.	b	11.	b
4.	b	12.	c
5.	a	13.	c
6.	a	14.	a
7.	b	15.	a
8.	b	16.	b

▶ CHAPTER 33

1.	e	17.	a, b
2.	b	18.	a, b, c
3.	a	19.	a
4.	d	20.	a
5.	a	21.	a
6.	b	22.	a, b
7.	a	23.	a, b
8.	a	24.	a
9.	d	25.	a
10.	b	26.	b
11.	b	27.	b
12.	a	28.	a, c, d
13.	d	29.	a
14.	a	30.	b, d
15.	a, b, c, d	31.	a
16.	a, b, c, d, e	32.	a, b, c, d

▶ CHAPTER 34

1.	d	**11.**	c	
2.	b	**12.**	d	
3.	b	**13.**	d	
4.	e	**14.**	c	
5.	b	**15.**	c	
6.	b	**16.**	d	
7.	c	**17.**	c	
8.	d	**18.**	a	
9.	e	**19.**	b	
10.	b	**20.**	b	

▶ CHAPTER 35

1.	b
2.	a
3.	c
4.	c
5.	b
6.	d
7.	b
8.	a

▶ CHAPTER 36

1.	d	**11.**	c
2.	d	**12.**	d
3.	b	**13.**	b
4.	d	**14.**	b
5.	a	**15.**	d
6.	b	**16.**	b
7.	d	**17.**	d
8.	a	**18.**	c
9.	b	**19.**	d
10.	c	**20.**	b

PART VI

Current Medical Education Questions

Current Medical Education Questions

▶ CHAPTER 1. INTEGRATIVE MEDICINE: BASIC PRINCIPLES

Learning Objectives:

a. define what is meant by "the healing system"

b. describe two research challenges in clinical research in integrative medicine

c. discuss the distinction between "healing" and "curing"

1-1. The expression of holism—i.e., the embodiment of the body/mind/spirit—is not a new paradigm. Which traditional medical models listed reflected this belief?

a. Greek medicine (Hippocratic era)
b. Roman medicine (Galenic era)
c. Heroic medicine (US ca. 1800)
d. Allopathic medicine (US ca. 1930s)

1-2. The term *integrative medicine* includes conventional biomedical treatments and alternative practices. What are the most distinguishing features that make it so different from conventional Western treatment?

a. it is a healing-oriented perspective
b. it includes complementary alternative medicine (CAM)
c. it focuses on the least invasive, least risky options for treatment
d. it is prevention oriented
e. all of the above

1-3. Approximately what percentage of the US population was actively using CAM in the survey performed by Eisenberg in 1993 and published in the *New England Journal of Medicine*?

a. 10%
b. 25%
c. 35%
d. 45%

1-4. Astin's article published in *JAMA* in 1998 revealed the reasons for CAM and integrative medical practices include the following

a. a wish to find a more holistic practitioner
b. the desire to get away from managed care
c. curiosity about the latest "fads" in medicine
d. a wish to find the cheapest health care possible

1-5. Knowledge can be acquired by many means. In the biomedical world, the strongest level of evidence of efficacy is felt to derive from the randomized controlled double-blind trial. For investigation of traditional medical systems such as acupuncture, pick the issues that may challenge this model in setting up a research protocol

a. individualized treatments for patients
b. unique definitions of disease and health states
c. multiple therapeutic interventions in one visit
d. all of the above

1-6. Pick options that would be interventions that reflect self-care for a busy physician

a. daily exercise
b. continuing to read an enjoyable book
c. occasional personal days for nonholiday family time
d. prioritizing medical work life to balance home and work time
e. managing professional opportunities that require work after hours
f. all of the above

1-7. Integrative medicine is a new specialty emerging in medicine.

a. true
b. false

1-8. Healing is a natural state of biological systems. In medical outcomes related to terminal illness, where prognosis is poor, measures to improve the quality of life represent a different kind of healing. Choose the options that reflect why

a. improvement in the quality of life during this time may help patients reflect on their relationship with their families and loved ones rather than exclusively seeing the illness as their identity
b. healing seeks to foster wholeness. Wholeness can occur within the realm of the mind–body experience as illness progresses. This can represent form of inner growth toward holism as the improvements in quality of life open up time for self-reflection
c. both a and b

1-9. Integration in medical care can be a healing-oriented perspective appropriate for all health care professionals.

a. true
b. false

1-10. Integrative practitioners embrace all forms of alternative therapy, regardless of whether data (from scientific trials) exist or not.

a. true
b. false

▶ **CHAPTER 2. PSYCHOSOCIAL DETERMINANTS OF HEALTH AND ILLNESS: REINTEGRATING MIND, BODY, AND SPIRIT**

Learning Objectives:

a. list and define the four quadrants of Wilbur's model as discussed in this chapter

b. give two examples of the evidence for the influence of socioeconomic factors on health outcomes

c. give an example of one study describing the connection between psychological factors and health outcomes

2-1. Wilber stated that if the world were reduced and descriptions were limited to the observable sciences,

a. the world would be empirically sound and prosperous

b. relationships would be based more on resources and agendas

c. the world would be devoid of depth and meaning

d. the world would be forced to place new focus on the importance of psychosocial variables in health

2-2. Modern mind–body beliefs are connected to Freud in which of the following ways?

a. unconscious motivations determine our interactions with medical professionals

b. unconscious processes are the root of evil

c. the id and superego influence the body, while the ego governs the mind

d. unconscious mental processes produce definite physiological symptoms

2-3. With regard to specific personality types and illnesses

a. the notion that specific personalities cause illnesses has no scientific support

b. the rheumatoid arthritis personality type was characterized as perfectionistic, compliant, subservient, restless, and angry

c. positive psychological states may influence health and well-being

d. all of the above

2-4. The relation between hostility and health can best be described by all of the following EXCEPT

a. hostility affects health only in those who are genetically predetermined for poor health

b. hostility is an independent risk factor for coronary heart disease

c. hostility leads to an increased risk for coronary heart disease (CHD), stroke, and heart attack

d. hostility is associated with behavioral risk factors

2-5. Delayed wound healing, prolonged infection, and increased production of proinflammatory cytokines are empirically related to

a. psychosocial stress

b. overmedication

c. poor nutritional habits

d. all of the above

2-6. Empirical studies have shown that the incidence of cardiac events has been directly related to all of the following EXCEPT

a. depression

b. hostility

c. self-esteem

d. hopelessness

2-7. In regard to cancer, which of the following has been shown

a. higher levels of depression predict higher mortality
b. anxiety and hostility in the family play a causal role
c. hopelessness and helplessness contribute to onset more than recovery
d. all of the above

2-8. Based on the findings of meta-analyses and randomized controlled trials, Astin et al. concluded that strong evidence exists to support the link between mind–body approaches in the treatment of all of the following EXCEPT

a. coronary artery disease
b. low back pain
c. headache
d. temporomandibular joint (TMJ) disorder

2-9. Using the quadrants from Wilber's model, the primary focus of treatment in the medical practice in the 19th and 20th centuries has been on the _____ quadrant(s), but in order to significantly influence health outcomes, more emphasis needs to be placed on the _____ quadrant(s)

a. upper left; upper right
b. lower right; upper left, lower left, and upper right
c. upper right; upper left, lower right, and lower left
d. lower right; upper left

2-10. The relation between lower socioeconomic status and poorer health can best be described as

a. curvilinear
b. nonexistent
c. reciprocal
d. linear

▶ CHAPTER 3. MIND–BODY MEDICINE

Learning Objectives:

a. define psychoneuroimmunology and give three examples of it at work in the human organism
b. define the concept of "allopathic load"
c. give three examples of mind–body therapies and define each

3-1. Self-regulation was first understood to be a stabilizing process governed by which body system?

a. immunologic
b. neuroendocrine
c. autonomic

3-2. In the stress response ("fight/flight"), corticotropin-releasing factor is produced by a specific neuroendocrine gland:

a. hypothalamus
b. pituitary
c. adrenal

3-3. Women may manifest a different biobehavioral response to stress. Which of the following hormones are *not* involved in this response?

a. adrenocorticotropic hormone (ACTH)
b. oxytocin
c. melatonin
d. cortisol

3-4. A new construct in the stress literature describes the pathophysiologic consequences of increased exposure to stress hormones. The term used for this phenomenon is

a. allostatic strain
b. accumulative stress
c. allostatic challenge
d. allostatic load

3-5. Individuals who have been classified alexithymic by psychoanalytically trained researchers are most likely to

a. internalize feelings
b. exaggerate feelings
c. symbolize distress
d. show an impoverished imaginary life

3-6. Tactile-kinesthetic stimulation is one way that a mother regulates her infant. In a study of premature babies, it contributed to

a. weight gain
b. increased head circumference
c. a alone
d. a and b

3-7. Individuals who somatize their distress are most likely to show which of the following characteristics?

a. high hypnotizability
b. low hypnotizability
c. parasympathetic dysregulation
d. sympathetic hyperactivity

3-8. The highest morbidity rates for individuals with depression have been found in the following condition

a. colon cancer
b. myocardial infarction
c. Parkinson's disease
d. breast cancer

3-9. Empirical research has found this mind–body therapy combined with cognitive behavioral therapy (CBT) to be effective in treating duodenal ulcers

a. guided imagery
b. hypnosis
c. mindfulness-based meditation

3-10. Which of the following is least emphasized by mind–body practitioners?

a. coping
b. transference
c. stress profiling
d. autonomic reactivity

▶ **CHAPTER 4. A NEW DEFINITION OF PATIENT-CENTERED MEDICINE**

Learning Objectives:

a. define the terms *antecedents*, *triggers*, and *mediators* as they are used in this chapter
b. give three examples of mediators
c. give three examples of common triggers of illness

4-1. The degree of pain and disability experienced by patients with osteoarthritis of the knees is most closely correlated with

a. quadriceps strength
b. radiographic abnormalities
c. sedimentation rate
d. duration of the disease

4-2. The mediators of illness for any patient may include

a. prostaglandins
b. reinforcement for staying ill
c. low self-efficacy
d. all of the above

4-3. Infection, connective tissue disease, coronary artery disease, diabetes, cancer, depression, obesity, and the physical impairments associated with aging are all strongly associated with

a. inflammation
b. trace mineral deficiency
c. hypogammaglobulinemia
d. slow intestinal transit

4-4. Sympathetic nervous system activation

a. may decrease intracellular magnesium
b. is inversely related to dietary magnesium
c. can increase irritability and noise sensitivity
d. all of the above

4-5. Disruption of the normal diurnal pattern of cortisol secretion among women with metastatic breast cancer is associated with

a. decreased natural killer (NK) cell cytotoxicity
b. shortened survival
c. divorce or widowhood
d. all of the above

4-6. The metabolic syndrome (syndrome X)

a. responds to a low glycemic index diet
b. responds to an increase in the ratio of polyunsaturated to saturated fat in the diet
c. affects almost a quarter of the US population
d. all of the above

4-7. Controlled studies have shown that inflammatory bowel disease, coronary artery disease, peripheral vascular disease, dysmenorrhea, cyclic mastalgia, cystic fibrosis, migraine headaches, bipolar disorder, and schizophrenia may be improved by

a. eating less meat and more whole grains
b. antioxidant supplementation
c. fish oil supplementation
d. treatment of food allergies

4-8. The patient's attempt to recognize triggers

a. is an impediment to scientific, evidence-based care
b. saves the physician time and allows him or her to concentrate on the scientific aspects of diagnosis and treatment
c. works best as a collaborative effort between patient and doctor
d. none of the above

4-9. Neurologic disorders of unkown cause, cerebellar degeneration, dermatitis herpetiformis, failure to thrive, pervasive developmental delay, inflammatory arthritis, and Sjögren's syndrome have been associated with

a. *Helicobacter pylori* infection
b. gluten intolerance
c. lactose intolerance
d. chronic giardiasis

4-10. Allergy to *Candida albicans*

a. has been implicated as a trigger for irritable bowel syndrome, urticaria, asthma, and chronic vaginitis
b. is unusual because *Candida* is part of the normal flora
c. is not associated with allergy to foodborne yeast

► CHAPTER 5. BOTANICAL MEDICINE: OVERVIEW

Learning Objectives:

a. describe two key points of the Dietary Supplement Health Education Act of 1994 (DSHEA)
b. give three examples of types of herbal formulations
c. list two reliable sources of information about herbal medicines

5-1. Botanical preparations have pharmacologic action, but because dosing is typically lower, they may have a lower prevalence of adverse effects.

a. true
b. false

5-2. A glycerine base liquid extract is an alternative to an alcohol base and can be used in those who have adverse reactions to alcohol.

a. true
b. false

5-3. In 1993, according to Eisenberg's telephone survey of 1500 respondents, botanical products were rated as the

a. most frequently used CAM modality
b. sixth most frequently used CAM modality
c. tenth most frequently used CAM modality
d. second most frequently used CAM modality

5-4. Which group of botanical practitioners is least likely to believe that whole plant products in liquid extracts and solid extracts may add unrecognized "active ingredients" of value to the recipient?

a. herbalists
b. physicians
c. traditional medical practitioners
d. naturopathists

5-5. Quality control in the United States is reliant on the manufacture's initiative.

a. true
b. false

5-6. Synergism in botanical pharmacology is one potential advantage of the right herbal preparation chosen as a medicinal alternative.

a. true
b. false

5-7. The Dietary Supplement Health and Education Act was created as a legislative mandate to define the use of botanical substances in the United States in 1964.

a. true
b. false

5-8. Glycerine-based liquid medications have shorter shelf lives than alcohol-based liquid extracts.

a. true
b. false

5-9. Adult doses can be modified for pediatric use, and all herbal remedies that are safe for adults are also safe for children.

a. true
b. false

5-10. Twenty-five percent of our current formulary is plant based today.

a. true
b. false

▶ **CHAPTER 6. ISSUES CONCERNING THE SAFETY OF STERBS AND PHYTOMEDICINAL PREPARATIONS**

Learning Objectives:

a. list three herbs known to have anticoagulant properties and how to use them safely

b. list two herbs that impact the hepatic metabolism of certain drugs and describe the mechanism of this interference

c. list four variables that will potentially impact both the safety and the efficacy of a botanical product

6-1. Adverse effects can be reported for a botanical substance, even though the product may be purchased over-the-counter.

a. true
b. false

6-2. Some botanical medicines should not be used when breast-feeding. Of the choices listed below, which one represents a safe botanical in lactation?

a. ginger
b. *Cascara sagrada* bark
c. chaste tree fruit
d. cinchona bark

6-3. Use of botanical substances and their safety are dependent on a number of variables, including which factors?

a. dosage
b. route of administration
c. the "biochemical individuality" of the patient
d. additive or antagonistic effects of other administered substances
e. all of the above

6-4. The DSHEA shifted the burden of proof of safety to the FDA and gave it authority to remove unsafe dietary supplements, only if the agency was able to prove they are unsafe in an administrative hearing that reviewed all case reports.

a. true
b. false

6-5. Which of the following safety classifications of botanical products proposed in McGuffin's book *Botanical Safety Handbook* describes herbs for which significant data exist to recommend the following labeling: "To be used only under the supervision of an expert qualified in the appropriate use of this substance"?

a. Class 2
b. Class 3
c. Class 1
d. Class 4

6-6. Attributing adverse effects to a specific botanical supplement includes verifying that the actual plant credited for the effect is not misidentified owing to poor quality control by the manufacturer. Another consideration is the adulteration of botanical products. Choose which substances have been found as adulterants in the recent past

a. heavy metals
b. steroids
c. nonsteroidal antiinflammatory agents
d. benzodiazepines
e. all of the above

6-7. Some plants are considered so toxic that they have been restricted from trade among the general public. These include which of the following?

a. *Aconitum napellus*
b. *Colchicum autumnale*
c. *Conium maculatum,*
d. *Datura* spp.
e. *Hyoscyamus niger*

6-8. Certain plants are recommended not to be used (as botanical supplements) during lactation. These include which of the following?

a. basil (*Ocimum basilicum*)
b. kava (*Piper methysticum*)
c. rhubarb root (*Rheum palmatum*)
d. ginger (*Zingiber officinale*)
e. senna (*Cassia senna*)

6-9. In studies of ginger, both mutagenic and antimutagenic properties have been suggested in in vitro studies.

a. true
b. false

6-10. Ginkgo is contraindicated in people with bleeding disorders owing to increased bleeding potential associated with regular use (6–12 months). Ginkgo should not be used at least how many hours before surgery?

a. 12 hours
b. 24 hours
c. 36 hours
d. 48 hours

▶ CHAPTER 7. INTEGRATIVE APPROACH TO NUTRITION

Learning Objectives:

a. describe the indications for and the components of the elimination diet approach

b. describe the indications for and rationale behind the low glycemic index diet

c. describe the indications for and the major components of the Dietary Approaches to Stop Hypertension (DASH) diet

7-1. Foods that are commonly excluded as part of an elimination diet protocol include which of the following?

a. wheat
b. dairy
c. oats
d. corn
e. lentils

7-2. An elimination diet can be useful in identifying food sensitivities that in certain cases can contribute to which of the following conditions?

a. atopic dermatitis
b. chronic rhinitis
c. migraine
d. irritable bowel syndrome
e. all of the above

7-3. The following are components of the standard "low glycemic diet"

a. 40% carbs/30% protein/30% fat
b. high polyunsaturated to saturated fatty acid ratio
c. high fiber intake
d. 20% carbs/40% protein/40% fats
e. high monounsaturated fatty acid intake

7-4. A low glycemic index diet can do which of the following?

a. lower blood lipids
b. decrease insulin sensitivity
c. increase insulinlike growth factors
d. reduce diabetes risk

7-5. Important elements of the DASH diet include which of the following?

a. under 4000 mg of sodium daily
b. increased fruit and vegetable intake
c. decreased sugar-containing beverages
d. increased whole grain products

7-6. The DASH diet had which of the following effects on serum lipids?

a. decreased total cholesterol
b. decreased LDL
c. decreased triglycerides
d. decreased HDL

7-7. The Paleolithic diet emphasizes which of the following?

a. increased animal protein from lean wild sources
b. decreased animal protein
c. elimination of dairy and grains
d. increase in low energy-density vegetable foods
e. all of the above

7-8. The specific carbohydrate diet (SCD) is low in

a. disaccharides
b. monosaccharides
c. polysaccharides

7-9. The SCD is used most often in which of the following conditions?

a. Crohn's disease
b. diabetes
c. gastroesophageal reflux disease
d. celiac disease

7-10. Spices that are believed to exhibit anti-inflammatory activity include which of the following?

a. ginger
b. rosemary
c. turmeric
d. garlic

▶ CHAPTER 8. CHIROPRACTIC AND OSTEOPATHIC CARE

Learning Objectives:

a. describe the training required to practice chiropractic currently in the United States

b. give two examples of clinical applications of chiropractic for conditions other than back pain

c. list the four basic principles of osteopathy

8-1. All of the following are true about chiropractic adjustments EXCEPT

a. most chiropractic adjustments are applied to synovial joints
b. chiropractic adjustments utilize a specific thrust which is low velocity and high amplitude
c. an adjustment restores range of motion to a joint
d. adjusting techniques that are low-force and nonforce are appropriate for children, pregnant patients, and patients with a risk of osteoporosis
e. chiropractic adjustments are specific and usually not painful

8-2. Chiropractic adjustment or subluxation complexes have all of the following effects EXCEPT

a. inhibit pain pathways at the spinal cord level of the adjustment
b. release endorphins and enkephalins at the spinal cord level of adjustment
c. reduce local inflammation
d. restore normal function to cranial nerves
e. cause reflexive relaxation of short spinal muscles at the level of adjustment

8-3. Chiropractic pediatric techniques might be effective for the following conditions EXCEPT

a. colic
b. difficult labor and delivery
c. otitis media
d. falls
e. anaphylactic shock

8-4. One challenge that researchers face in chiropractic research is

a. finding a suitable sham treatment
b. developing adjusting protocols that can be duplicated appropriately from patient to patient
c. developing a large enough sample size
d. developing intertester reliability
e. all of the above

8-5. The most serious risk of cervical manipulation is

a. headache
b. strain
c. cerebrovascular accident (CVA)
d. fracture

8-6. The most serious risk of lumbar manipulation is

a. strain
b. disc herniation
c. cauda equina syndrome
d. stenosis

8-7. The major principles of osteopathy include all of the following except

a. the body is a unit designed to move
b. nerve function is more important than circulation in maintaining health
c. structure and function are reciprocally related by motion
d. the body possesses self healing and regulatory mechanisms

8-8. Counterstrain is an osteopathic technique that involves passive lengthening of contracted muscles while holding tender points on muscle, ligament, or tendon.

a. true
b. false

8-9. Chiropractic would be an appropriate treatment for all of the following EXCEPT

a. cervical whiplash
b. lumbar sprain/strain
c. repetitive stress injuries
d. torn rotator cuff
e. headaches

8-10. The trend in the research shows that spinal manipulation done with great skill can improve the symptoms of herniated lumbar discs, therefore it is a viable alternative to surgery.

a. true
b. false

▶ CHAPTER 9. ACUPUNCTURE AND EAST ASIAN MEDICINE

Learning Objectives:

a. give three examples of conditions for which the use of acupuncture is strongly supported by clinical trials

b. define what is meant by the term *kanbing* and how the process of diagnosis in East Asian medicine differs from the process in Western medicine

c. list three examples of manual techniques other than needling used in East Asian medicine for stimulation of a healing response

9-1. Acupuncture needles generally require a minimum insertion depth of

a. 1/4 inch
b. 1 inch
c. 2 inches

9-2. *de Qi* is the Chinese term that describes

a. the organ that controls digestion in the body
b. the sensation at a point if it has been needled successfully
c. the interaction between the body fluids and the organs
d. the process of palpation for tender points

9-3. Proposed mechanisms for acupuncture's effect from a Western biomedicine perspective include

a. endorphin release
b. mast cell stimulation
c. connective tissue fiber winding
d. all of the above

9-4. Conditions for which the 1997 NIH Consensus Panel determined acupuncture to be "promising" included which of the following?

a. postoperative nausea
b. postoperative dental pain
c. fibromyalgia
d. chemotherapy-induced nausea
e. cancer pain

9-5. Studies of acupuncture for labor have demonstrated which of the following to be true?

a. acupuncture can shorten the active phase of labor
b. acupuncture reduces the incidence of cesarean section
c. acupuncture is effective in reducing pain during labor
d. acupuncture is effective in inducing post-dates labor

9-6. Conditions for which acupuncture was assessed as "may be helpful" in the 1997 NIH Consensus statement include

a. menstrual pain
b. chronic fatigue syndrome
c. depression
d. osteoarthritis
e. asthma

9-7. *Kanbing* means

a. the practitioner and patient look at the patient's problem together
b. the practitioner and patient breathe together during pulse taking
c. the radial pulse is rapid
d. the patient cannot fully flex their fingers

9-8. Pain is an expression of

a. interruption in free flow
b. imbalance in elements
c. deficiency of the blood
d. congestion in the liver

9-9. Acupuncture is often used in conjunction with

a. gua sha or cupping
b. direct or indirect moxibustion
c. herbal medicine and dietary recommendations
d. all of the above

9-10. The concept of Qi represents both form and function and corresponds to early Western medicine's

a. pneuma
b. yellow bile
c. blood
d. vitalism

▶ CHAPTER 10. AYURVEDIC MEDICINE

Learning Objectives:

a. describe three qualities associated with each of the doshas
b. list and describe the five major components of the Ayurvedic approach
c. define and describe the term *Panchakarma*

10-1. The word *Ayurveda* can be defined as

a. natural living
b. practice of yoga
c. life science or life knowledge
d. vegetarianism

10-2. Life according to Ayurveda is the harmonious blending of these three

a. body, mind, and soul
b. herbs, meditation, and yoga
c. childhood, youth, and old age
d. body, mind, and nutrition

10-3. Which of the following is a unique feature of Ayurveda?

a. administering the whole plant herbal drug in treatment
b. symptomatic approach to treatment
c. administering the active principle of the herbs (standardized extracts)
d. treating the patients without using herbs

10-4. Which dosha represents the principle of movement in the body?

a. vata
b. pitta
c. kapha
d. dhatu

10-5. Characteristics of Vata dosha include

a. hot and heavy
b. cold and light
c. heavy and moist
d. moist and sour

10-6. Pitta in the body is responsible for this function

a. voluntary and involuntary movements
b. biotransformation
c. movement of ovum to the womb
d. lubrication

10-7. Kapha dosha is predominantly located in this part of the body

a. upper part of the trunk
b. middle part of the trunk
c. lower part of the trunk
d. extremities

10-8. The following is an example of excessive (aggravated) Kapha dosha

a. skin rashes
b. arthritis
c. anxiety
d. mucus expectoration

10-9. The goal of pancha karma is to

a. eliminate toxins from the body
b. restoration of the body tissues
c. improvement of mental functions
d. all of the above

10-10. One of the first herbal treatments used for hypertension (shonita dushti) was

a. snuhi (*Euphoria nerifolia*)
b. shigru (*Moringa olifera*)
c. sarpagandha (*Rauwolfia serpentine*)
d. none of the above

▶ **CHAPTER 11. MOVEMENT AND BODY-CENTERED THERAPIES**

Learning Objectives:

a. discuss the evidence from the medical literature regarding the therapeutic benefits of Hatha yoga
b. list and describe four different massage techniques
c. discuss the evidence for two medical applications of Tai Chi and Qigong

11-1. Tai chi has shown evidence-based benefit for

a. arthritis and cardiovascular problems
b. asthma and colds
c. edema and urinary retention
d. infertility and repeated miscarriage

11-2. Qigong exercises may contribute to

a. increased bone mass
b. improved blood circulation
c. improved eyesight
d. all of the above

11-3. The *asanas* are the postures in Hatha yoga.

a. true
b. false

11-4. The postures of Hatha yoga involve
1. standing poses
2. seated poses and forward bending
3. inversions
4. backbends

a. 1 and 3
b. 2 and 4
c. 4
d. all of the above

11-5. Clinical research on the potential usefulness of Hatha yoga is available in the areas of
1. asthma
2. hypertension
3. osteoarthritis
4. headaches

a. 1 is true
b. 1 and 3 are true
c. 4 is true
d. all are true

11-6. A Hatha yoga intervention was shown to be useful for carpal tunnel syndrome in a randomized controlled clinical trial published in 1998 in the *Journal of the American Medical Association*.

a. true
b. false

11-7. Mindfulness-based stress reduction (MBSR) has been shown to have a positive influence on the rate of skin clearing in patients with moderate to severe psoriasis undergoing phototherapy (UVB) and photochemotherapy (PUVA).

a. true
b. false

11-8. The Feldenkreis method is based on the assumption that habitual movements and postures represent a disruption in the nervous system and that gentle movement and manipulation can replace old patterns of movement with new ones.

a. true
b. false

11-9. Yoga teachers who offer therapeutic yoga classes
1. are required to have certification as a yoga teacher
2. are required to be licensed healthcare providers
3. usually work in a hospital or clinical setting

a. 1 is true
b. 2 is true
c. 2 and 3 are true
d. none are true

11-10. Dean Ornish has developed a program of cardiac rehabilitation that has been shown through several large clinical studies to be an effective strategy to reverse coronary artery disease. This program includes yoga.

a. true
b. false

▶ CHAPTER 12. HOMEOPATHY

Learning Objectives:

a. define the "Law of Similars"

b. list two common homeopathic remedies for treatment of trauma and two for treatment of otitis in children, and give two characteristics for each of these remedies

c. discuss the distinction between the "polypharmacy" approach to homeopathy and the "classical" approach

12-1. Homeopathy is based on the following theoretical principles

a. small doses, signatures, energy meridians
b. small doses, organ affinities, channeling
c. Principle of Similars, Provings, small doses
d. Principle of Similars, Hering's Law, Avogadro's Principle

12-2. Homeopathic concentration 30C means that the substance was diluted

a. 30 times
b. 10^{-3} times
c. 10^{-30} times
d. 10^{-60} times

12-3. The homeopathic term *proving* describes

a. a process of discovering medicinal characteristics of substances by administering them in homeopathic concentrations to sensitive healthy volunteers following the double-blinded placebo-controlled protocol
b. a process of quality control that involves administration of homeopathic remedies to animals following the double-blinded placebo-controlled protocol
c. a process of providing research data to prove that homeopathy works

12-4. Key elements of the homeopathic evaluation include

a. mental/emotional symptoms
b. sensation, location, direction
c. modalities, concomitant symptoms
d. intensity, duration, onset, chronological sequence of symptoms
e. all of the above

12-5. According to homeopathic theory, a *true acute* is defined as

a. a new, never before experienced, usually self-limiting condition

b. an exacerbation of a chronic condition that presents with similar but more severe symptoms

c. both

d. neither

12-6. The most important homeopathic remedy for treatment of musculoskeletal trauma is:

a. *Arnica montana*

b. *Aconitum napellis*

c. belladonna

d. *Spongia*

12-7. Patients who can benefit from *Arnica*

a. frequently become very anxious and seek company

b. frequently become restless and feel better from movement

c. frequently think that there is nothing wrong with them and refuse help

d. all of the above

e. none of the above

12-8. Choose remedies that are matched correctly with specific conditions

a. aconite: trauma accompanied by great fright or terror

b. cantharis: severe (second- and third-degree) burns; severe, horrible burning much improved by cold applications

c. hypericum: injuries to areas with a high concentration of pain receptors—fingers, genitalia, tongue; crushing injuries to fingertips

d. all of the above

12-9. Symptoms that warrant use of *Aconitum* in treatment of croup are

a. sudden onset in the first 24 hours of illness accompanied by severe fear and restlessness

b. glassy eyes with enlarged pupils

c. patient feel better when lying still

d. all of the above

12-10. Children with flu or common cold may benefit from belladonna if they present with

a. rapid onset and extremely high fever

b. flushed, red, hot face, but hands and/or feet are cold

c. delirious state

d. all of the above

▶ CHAPTER 13. PHYSICAL ACTIVITY AND EXERCISE

Learning Objectives:

a. describe the evidence for the role of exercise in prevention and treatment of three disease conditions

b. discuss a strategy for safely recommending exercise for patients over 55 years old

c. summarize the current recommendations regarding exercise for children and adolescents

13-1. Research has demonstrated that physical activity decreases the risk of type 1 and type 2 diabetes.

a. true

b. false

13-2. The public health recommendations for physical activity encourage 30 minutes of continuously performed intense physical activity.

a. true

b. false

13-3. Parents should wait until their child is at least 2 years of age before engaging them in physical exercise-directed activities.

a. true
b. false

13-4. The greatest risk factor for adult overweight and obesity is adolescent overweight and obesity.

a. true
b. false

13-5. All individuals >50 years of age should undergo formalized testing before beginning any exercise program.

a. true
b. false

13-6. Seniors should be encouraged to slowly warm-up and cool-down, avoiding rapid changes in body temperature that may place undue stress on the cardiovascular system.

a. true
b. false

13-7. The four elements of the traditional exercise prescription include: frequency, intensity, type, and tempo (FITT).

a. true
b. false

13-8. An inverse dose-response relationship has been suggested to exist for physical activity and mild to moderate depression.

a. true
b. false

13-9. The exact mechanism by which physical activity and exercise affects depression has been shown to be release of ß-endorphins.

a. true
b. false

13-10. All forms of aerobic conditioning have been demonstrated to have therapeutic benefits in osteoporosis.

a. true
b. false

▶ CHAPTER 14. SPIRITUALITY AND HEALTH

Learning Objectives:

a. give two examples of strategies for taking a spiritual history

b. list two controversies regarding the role of physicians in discussing spiritual issues with patients

c. give three examples of evidence from the literature regarding the impact of prayer and/or "nonlocal healing" on specific health conditions

14-1. The Medicine Wheel is

a. a token of payment for health care
b. a pantheistic icon
c. a symbol of life and spirit
d. a sought-after icon believed to be an aphrodisiac

14-2. An inextricable relationship between all aspects of the universe: physical, psychical, and spiritual, has been supported by:

a. theories of quantum physics
b. the *Philosophy of Universal Intersections*
c. the modern medical school curriculum
d. a recently developed school of psychotherapy known as Relationship-Centered Care

14-3. In the typical modern-day physician visit, the patient may be restricted from involvement in health care choices because of

a. the failure of the patient and physician to communicate about the patient's views
b. certain concerns about the cost of care and national health care reimbursement
c. both lack of communication and cost considerations
d. none of the above

14-4. Spirituality can be broadly defined as being

a. intrapersonal
b. an inherent aspect of every human being
c. that domain in which values and meaning exist
d. all of these

14-5. Religion is a body of beliefs and practices that are defined by a community or society and allied with a set of doctrines and practices to which its adherents mutually subscribe, and is therefore more

a. relativistic
b. incapable of definition
c. external and interpersonal
d. never highly personal

14-6. Religious practices offer substantial quality-of-life benefits to their practitioners and

a. decreased hospital stays
b. improved longevity
c. decreased all-cause mortality and morbidity
d. all of these

14-7. Four approaches to eliciting a spiritual history are mentioned. Which one of these is *not* included?

a. Three Questions
b. FICA
c. HELP
d. SPIRITual History

14-8. It can be difficult to initiate religious discussions or pray with patients because

a. patients cannot articulate well
b. there is a plurality and heterogeneity of religious beliefs
c. religion is embarrassing to both patients and physicians
d. religion is not relevant to patient care

14-9. Some trained chaplains have expressed a belief that

a. few patients have strong spiritual beliefs, so spiritual matters are unimportant in medical care
b. physicians should never take a spiritual history under any circumstance
c. physicians may not possess the requisite interpersonal and intrapersonal skills to facilitate conversations in the religious domain
d. every physician should take a complete spiritual history on every initial patient visit

14-10. Family practice physicians have identified the following barriers to addressing religion and spirituality in health care with patients

a. inadequate time to spend discussing such matters
b. inadequate training
c. difficulty in patient identification in relation to religious issues
d. all of the above

► CHAPTER 15. INFORMATICS AND INTEGRATIVE MEDICINE

Learning Objectives:

a. list three criteria that are useful in assessing the credibility of an integrative medicine–oriented Website

b. name three nonproprietary databases that can be useful in searching for information on integrative medicine

c. define what is meant by a MEsH term

15-1. The best way to search MEDLINE is to do a keyword search.

a. true
b. false

15-2. A useful Website for the independent evaluation of herbal and dietary supplements is

a. Herbmed
b. Consumerlab.com
c. Altmedex
d. Natural Medicines Comprehensive Database

15-3. The MeSH heading *complementary therapies* provides complete coverage of the CM literature in MEDLINE.

a. true
b. false

15-4. A MEDLINE search will generally retrieve which percentage of randomized controlled trials on a given topic?

a. 25%
b. 50%
c. 90%

15-5. It is important to explode a MeSH heading because articles in MEDLINE are indexed by using the most specific MeSH term that applies.

a. true
b. false

15-6. Important criteria for evaluating Websites include all except

a. the currency of the information
b. the publishing organization
c. the size of the Website
d. the design of the Website

15-7. The Cochrane Library is a valuable resource for CM searching because it covers many CM sources that are not indexed in MEDLINE.

a. true
b. false

15-8. Good sources for searching mind–body medicine include all of the following except

a. MEDLINE
b. CINAHL
c. HealthStar
d. PsychLit

15-9. MEDLINE searching alone for CM topics is inadequate because

a. it does not cover the international literature
b. it does not cover all the CM journals
c. it has no MeSH headings for CM topics

15-10. A free evidence-based database on herbal medicine is provided by

a. American Botanical Council
b. Herb Research Foundation
c. HerbMed
d. Natural Medicine Comprehensive Database

► CHAPTER 16. SELECTED ISSUES IN ENVIRONMENTAL MEDICINE

Learning Objectives:

a. define "sick building syndrome" and list three factors that may predispose patients to its development

b. list and describe three strategies for access to safe and healthy drinking water

c. list three health conditions potentially exacerbated by air pollution

16-1. Studies suggest that health benefits of drinking adequate amounts of clean water may include which of the following?

a. a decrease in the relative risk of fatal coronary heart disease in humans
b. a protective association between zinc and magnesium content found in drinking water and type 2 diabetes
c. a decreased severity of neuropathology in Alzheimer's disease in animal models
d. all of the above

16-2. Waterborne pathogen resistance to multiple antibiotics may be a result of which of the following?

a. source water contamination by antibiotics and bioactive chemicals used in the human population
b. unregulated and massive use of antibiotics in aquaculture and agriculture
c. gene exchange of antibiotic resistance factors by biofilms present in water system processing tanks
d. all of the above

16-3. While a number of methods are employed to assure drinking water purity, chlorine remains the most common and important drinking water disinfectant.

a. true
b. false

16-4. All bottled waters are subject to federal standards including regulatory requirements for maximum contaminant levels (MCLs) and good manufacturing practices.

a. true
b. false

16-5. Peak ozone levels usually occur when weather is

a. cool, cloudy
b. hot, muggy
c. cold, dry
d. rainy

16-6. Diseases associated with air pollution include

a. heart disease
b. stroke
c. lung cancer
d. rhinoconjunctivitis

16-7. HEPA (high-efficiency particulate air) filters are of the mechanical filter type.

a. true
b. false

16-8. Risk factors for sick building syndrome include all of the following except

a. low-paying job category
b. atopy
c. male sex
d. use of a video display terminal

16-9. Characteristics of the environment in sick building syndrome include

a. smoking
b. high room temperatures
c. low-frequency noise
d. low-frequency fluorescent lamps
e. all of the above

16-10. Abnormalities of balance, color vision, and verbal recall have been shown in the literature to be associated with exposure to

a. benzene
b. formaldehyde
c. perchloroethylene
d. ozone

▶ **CHAPTER 17. INTEGRATIVE APPROACH TO ALLERGY**

Learning Objectives:

a. describe the use of herbal medicines and supplements in the integrative treatment of allergic rhinitis
b. discuss the relationship between testing for food allergies using blood tests, skin tests, and elimination trials
c. describe three important aspects of the integrative approach to the treatment of multiple chemical sensitivities

17-1. Which of the following mast cell–stabilizing botanicals has had good results in treating allergic rhinitis, and therefore may be useful in treating chronic urticaria?

a. licorice
b. echinacea
c. quercetin
d. milkweed

17-2. True food allergies are associated with which one of the following immunoglobulins?

a. IgE
b. IgG
c. IgA
d. IgM

17-3. Tree pollens cross react with which of the following foods?

a. apples
b. bananas
c. turkey
d. cantaloupe

17-4. What proportion of infants demonstrate an adverse food reaction?

a. 1/3
b. 1/2
c. 3/4

17-5. Which childhood allergies are not usually outgrown and persist into adulthood?

a. peanut
b. wheat
c. dairy
d. tree nuts

17-6. A positive skin test only confirms the presence of allergen-specific IgE in the bloodstream—it never confirms a food allergy.

a. true
b. false

17-7. Only 40% of individuals with a positive skin test to a food allergen will actually manifest a symptom when that food is ingested.

a. true
b. false

17-8. Which of the following are considered hypoallergenic foods?

a. lamb
b. chicken
c. almonds
d. potatoes
e. rice
f. mango

17-9. Extracts of stinging nettles possess antihistaminic properties.

a. true
b. false

17-10. Enteric-coated capsules of peppermint oil can be helpful for abdominal pain related to bowel spasms, but may exacerbate gastroesophageal reflux.

a. true
b. false

► CHAPTER 18. INTEGRATIVE APPROACH TO CARDIOVASCULAR HEALTH

Learning Objectives:

a. describe the Mediterranean diet and discuss its impact on cardiovascular disease.

b. discuss the current controversy regarding the impact of alcohol consumption on cardiovascular disease risk

c. list three interventions which have been shown to be of benefit in outcomes for patients with heart disease

18-1. The five major risk factors for coronary artery disease include all of the following except

a. abnormal lipids
b. cigarette smoking
c. alcohol use
d. obesity
e. diabetes mellitus
f. sedentary lifestyle

18-2. Which of the following interventions have been shown to significantly affect outcome in patients with stable, chronic coronary artery disease?

a. coronary artery balloon angioplasty
b. statin medications
c. smoking cessation
d. coronary artery stenting
e. weight loss

18-3. Which of the following correlates more closely with coronary artery disease risk?

a. total dietary fat
b. saturated animal fat

18-4. Monounsaturated fat, associated with a lower risk of coronary heart disease, is found in which of the following sources?

a. tree nuts
b. olive oil
c. soybean oil
d. avocados
e. flaxseed oil

18-5. The Lyon Diet Heart Study showed a 70% improvement in outcomes using a diet high in which of the following?

a. alpha-linolenic acid
b. omega-3 fatty acids
c. monounsaturated fats
d. *trans*-fatty acids

18-6. Food sources of omega-3 fatty acids include

a. deep sea fish
b. flaxseed oil
c. evening primrose oil
d. walnuts
e. avocado

18-7. The number of excess deaths that occur yearly due to sedentary lifestyle is believed to be approximately

a. 10,000
b. 50,000
c. 200,000

18-8. The metabolic impact of regular exercise includes which of the following?

a. improved carbohydrate metabolism
b. decreased HDL-C
c. favorable changes in LDL particle size
d. improved plasma insulin levels

18-9. The "atherogenic metabolic triad" includes which of the following?

a. hyperinsulinemia
b. small, dense LDL particles
c. hyperapolipoproteinemia B
d. increased homocysteine levels

18-10. Severe depression may increase the risk of death from coronary disease by a factor of

a. 2–4
b. 4–6
c. 8–10

▶ CHAPTER 19. INTEGRATIVE APPROACH TO CHRONIC FATIGUE SYNDROME

Learning Objectives:

a. give three examples of nutritional interventions commonly used in the integrative approach to CFS

b. discuss the evidence regarding the use of mind–body therapies for patients with CFS

c. discuss the pros and cons of exercise for patients with CFS and the current recommendations regarding exercise for this population

19-1. The CDC 1994 case definition for CFS is the definition most commonly used in research investigations of this condition.

a. true
b. false

19-2. CFS is more common in men than women.

a. true
b. false

19-3. Nutritional deficiency is a common finding in patients with CFS.

a. true
b. false

19-4. Which of the following has not been associated with the pathophysiology of CFS?

a. diet
b. preexisting insomnia
c. celiac disease
d. cultural influences

19-5. Coenzyme Q10 has been shown to dramatically improve symptoms in patients with CFS.

a. true
b. false

19-6. Is CFS a disease or a syndrome?

a. CFS is a disease
b. CFS is a syndrome
c. there is not enough evidence to determine

19-7. Patients presenting with CFS must be treated with what in mind?

a. an eye toward excluding fibromyalgia and other similar syndromes before making a diagnosis of CFS
b. making sure the patient has the social support system necessary to cope with the condition
c. usefulness of psychiatric interventions
d. all of the above

19-8. Fatigue is the characteristic symptom of CFS, but its duration must be

a. less than 6 months
b. more than 12 months
c. more than 6 months
d. duration is not an issue

19-9. Chinese medicine generally views CFS as a disorder of what?

a. liver Qi stagnation
b. heart and kidney dampness
c. overactive spleen function

19-10. Pathophysiology of CFS is often attributed to

a. Epstein-Barr virus
b. immune dysfunction
c. endocrine dysfunction
d. all of the above

► CHAPTER 20. INTEGRATIVE APPROACH TO ENDOCRINOLOGY

Learning Objectives:

a. give three examples of botanical medicines that may be of benefit for patients with diabetes

b. discuss the use of herbal medicines and nutritional supplements in the treatment of hypothyroidism

c. give three examples of the integrative approach to symptom management in hyperthyroidism

20-1. Which of the following statements is most accurate?

a. small studies of short duration have shown that vanadyl sulfate has no beneficial effect in patients with diabetes

b. large randomized controlled trials have found that vanadium is effective for reducing fasting glucose and HbA_{1c} levels

c. studies of vanadyl sulfate have been primarily discontinued due to significant toxicity concerns

d. small studies of short duration have shown that vanadyl sulfate has beneficial effects in patients with diabetes

20-2. Which of the following statements is most accurate?

a. refined grains contain substantially more dietary fiber and magnesium than whole grains

b. the Nurses' Health Study found that a high cereal fiber intake was associated with increased risk of diabetes

c. psyllium has been shown to reduce postprandial glucose levels and reduce fasting blood glucose

d. researchers have repeatedly failed to find an inverse association between diabetes and high intake of whole grains

20-3. Which of the following statements are true?

a. fish oil may hasten the progression of diabetic retinopathy

b. fish oil improves nerve conduction velocity in animal studies

c. fish oil elevated triglycerides in diabetics with hyperlipidemia

d. fish oil may help prevent diabetic neuropathy

20-4. Preliminary studies suggest that which of the following has hypoglycemic activity?

a. bitter melon

b. evening primrose oil

c. cayenne

d. gymnema

20-5. There are over 100 clinical trials on homeopathic remedies for the treatment of diabetes in the peer-reviewed literature.

a. true

b. false

20-6. Which of the following deficiencies can lead to hypothyroidism?

a. iron

b. selenium

c. chromium

d. iodine

20-7. Oral administration of bugleweed in animals studies noted

a. reduction in TSH only

b. reduction in T_3 only

c. reduction in T_4 only

d. no reduction in TSH, T_3 or T_4

20-8. Which of the following herbs was traditionally used for tachycardia and palpitations?

a. motherwort

b. kelp

c. bilberry

d. fenugreek

20-9. Which of the following statements is most accurate about bilberry?

a. two small double-blind, placebo-controlled studies have shown improved ophthalmoscopic patterns in patients with diabetic retinopathy

b. clinical trials have been conducted on products standardized to contain 2.5% bilberry glucosides

c. the antioxidant and vascular stabilizing activity of bilberry extract would make it a poor choice for diabetics

d. the majority of research on bilberry has been conducted on the leaf, not the fruit.

20-10. The German Commission E recognized motherwort for

a. symptomatic relief of hyperthyroidism

b. congestive heart failure

c. cardiac disorders associated with anxiety

d. primary treatment of hyperthyroidism

▶ CHAPTER 21. INTEGRATIVE APPROACH TO THE GASTROINTESTINAL SYSTEM

Learning Objectives:

a. discuss the relationship between intestinal flora and systemic inflammation

b. describe three aspects of the integrative approach to management of inflammatory bowel disease

c. discuss the integrative approach to the treatment of irritable bowel syndrome

21-1. Intestinal dysbiosis is

a. another name for irritable bowel syndrome

b. a serious infection with pathogenic bacteria

c. a disruption in the normal relationship between the human host and the indigenous gut flora

d. none of the above

21-2. Milk-derived lactoferrins

a. are used by bacteria to support their growth

b. slow intestinal transit

c. starve bacteria of iron needed for growth

d. improve zinc absorption

21-3. Intestinal motility is inhibited by

a. magnesium

b. fish oils

c. dopaminergic neurons

d. serotonergic neurons

21-4. Acid-lowering drugs

a. permit bacterial overgrowth in the stomach

b. increase susceptibility to intestinal pathogens

c. may cause vitamin B_{12} malabsorption

d. all of the above

21-5. Which of the following probiotics is not found as part of the normal indigenous flora?

a. *Lactobacillus* GG

b. *Lactobacillus plantarum*

c. *Saccharomyces boulardii*

d. *Bifidobacterium brevis*

21-6. Which of the following is true concerning the small intestinal permeability to intact protein?

a. the small bowel mucosa is totally impermeable to dietary protein; only small peptides or amino acids are absorbed

b. macrophages transport dietary protein across the mucosal lining by interrupting the basement membrane

c. cellular adhesion molecules permit protein transport through the paracellular pathway

d. intact protein is normally transported across enterocytes by endocytosis

21-7. Glutamine has been shown to improve

a. colonic motility

b. abnormal small intestinal permeability

c. symptoms of gastroesophageal reflux disease

d. elimination of gallstones from the gallbladder

21-8. The psychosocial intervention with the greatest evidence for benefit among patients with inflammatory bowel disease is

a. hypnotherapy
b. individualized self-management training
c. support groups
d. cognitive behavior therapy

21-9. The following natural products have been shown helpful in the control of inflammation in ulcerative colitis

a. fish oils
b. boswellia
c. aloe vera mucopolysaccharides
d. all of the above

21-10. Which of the following was found in a controlled trial of traditional Chinese medicinal herbs for patients with irritable bowel syndrome?

a. formulations individualized for each patient were the only ones that produced sustained symptom reduction after the treatment was discontinued
b. formulations individualized for each patient produced a greater degree of symptom relief than a standardized generic bowel formula
c. the placebo response rate was so high that the potential benefits of any type of herbal formula could not be assessed
d. side effects of the herbal treatment were greater than the benefits

▶ CHAPTER 22. INTEGRATIVE APPROACH TO NEUROLOGY

Learning Objectives:

a. discuss the use of herbs and supplements in the treatment and prevention of Alzheimer's disease

b. list three aspects of the integrative approach to multiple sclerosis

c. discuss one current theory regarding the etiology of Parkinson's disease and one strategy for prevention from the integrative perspective

22-1. Which of the following statements in regard to integrative strategies to treat Alzheimer's disease is not true?

a. antioxidants are included in the integrative approach to treating Alzheimer's disease
b. hormone replacement therapy is a proven effective treatment for Alzheimer's disease
c. lipid lowering strategies may reduce the risk of Alzheimer's disease
d. neuroprotective agents are currently being explored as possible adjuncts to treatment of Alzheimer's disease

22-2. Which antioxidant has demonstrated possible efficacy in delaying the progression of Alzheimer's disease?

a. vitamin C
b. vitamin B_{12}
c. vitamin E
d. glutathione

22-3. Which fatty acid is diminished in the neuronal membranes of Alzheimer's patients?

a. EPA
b. cholesterol
c. linoleic acid
d. DHA

22-4. Which of the following environmental factors has not been linked to a risk of Parkinson's disease?

a. rural living
b. drinking well water
c. exposure to pesticides
d. consumption of a high-fat Western-diet

22-5. Which of the following supplements has been best studied as a neuroprotective agent in Parkinson's disease?

a. lipoic acid
b. vitamin E
c. vitamin C
d. glutathione

22-6. Which of the following explanations may account for the lack of efficacy of vitamin E in Parkinson's disease?

a. vitamin E may have limited access across the blood–brain barrier to increase brain vitamin E levels

b. vitamin E can be converted to a pro-oxidant in diseased tissue

c. higher doses of vitamin E need to be used to observe a beneficial effect

d. vitamin E may not be effective once disease symptoms become overtly manifested

22-7. Coenzyme Q10 therapy has recently been found to be beneficial in improving symptoms of Parkinson's disease in multicenter studies.

a. true
b. false

22-8. Recent epidemiologic data suggest a strong correlation between dental amalgams and multiple sclerosis

a. true
b. false

22-9. Which two herbs have been proposed as possible useful alternative therapies in the management of multiple sclerosis?

a. St. John's wort and *Ginkgo biloba*
b. echinacea and goldenseal
c. curcumin and tripterygium
d. ginseng and Ginkgo

22-10. What is the correct proposed mechanism for how mind–body therapies may be helpful in reducing multiple sclerosis relapses?

a. increased levels of endorphins which may be immunosuppressive

b. reduction of corticotropin-releasing factor (CRF)

c. upregulation of serotinergic neurotransmission

d. reduced macrophage accumulation at the site of injury

▶ CHAPTER 23. INTEGRATIVE APPROACH TO ONCOLOGY

Learning Objectives:

a. discuss the pros and cons of antioxidant use for patients with cancer

b. list three nutritional strategies for cancer prevention and treatment

c. describe the evidence for and against mind–body therapies for patients with cancer

23-1. A landmark Finnish trial supplementing beta-carotene in adults with high risk for lung cancer demonstrated

a. no benefit

b. 90% reduction in subsequent occurrence of small-cell lung cancer

c. an increase in lung cancer

d. a higher risk of jaundice in those receiving beta-carotene

23-2. Xerostomia due to radiation has been demonstrated

a. to be reduced by beta-carotene

b. to be effectively treated by acupuncture

c. to be reduced by a modified high-pH diet

d. to be treatable with ginger

23-3. Acupuncture for nausea and vomiting due to chemotherapy

a. has no risk for complications

b. has been considered clearly effective by an NIH Consensus Development Panel on acupuncture

c. should be routinely prescribed for chemotherapy patients

d. is a substitute for antiemetic drug therapy

23-4. One mushroom not known to have anticancer properties is

a. *Lentinus edodes* (shiitake)
b. *Ganoderma lucidum* (reishi)
c. *Tuber magnatum* (white truffle)
d. *Grifola frondosa* (maitake)

23-5. Cyclooxygenase inhibiting activity is found in

a. red raspberry
b. curcumin
c. burdock
d. isatis

23-6. Which of the following vitamins have the most in vitro research supporting their effectiveness against cancer

a. vitamin B_{12} (cyanobalamin)
b. vitamin K_1 (phylloquinone)
c. vitamin D_3 (1,25-hydroxycholecalciferol)
d. vitamin B_1 (thiamine)

23-7. There are studies showing improved survival for which of the following cancers with supportive psychotherapeutic interventions?

a. breast cancer
b. sarcoma
c. hepatocarcinoma
d. small-cell lung cancer

23-8. Which of the following substance(s) are contraindicated in estrogen positive breast cancer?

a. bovine cartilage
b. red clover (*Trifolium pratense* L.)
c. American ginseng (*Panax quinquefolius* L.)
d. dang guai (*Angelica sinensis*)
e. melatonin

23-9. The following botanical ingredients have immunostimulatory properties

a. flavonoids
b. polysaccharides
c. aromatic oils
d. trace metals

23-10. Phytoestrogens

a. are found in soy products
b. have not been shown to prevent breast cancer
c. can treat estrogen positive breast cancer

▶ CHAPTER 24. INTEGRATIVE APPROACH TO OSTEOPOROSIS

Learning Objectives:

a. list five nutritional supplements that should be part of the integrative approach to osteoporosis
b. discuss three food or drink items to be avoided and three to be included to help in prevention of bone loss
c. discuss the role of exercise and mind–body therapies in prevention and treatment of osteoporosis and the proposed mechanism for each

24-1. All of the following are functions of bone except

a. structural support
b. metabolize nutrients
c. nutrient reservoir
d. growth stimulation

24-2. All of the following are true about osteoclasts except

a. it is a multinucleated giant cell derived from a monocyte
b. they function best in a basic environment
c. they are activated by macrophage colony-stimulating factor, cytokines, prostaglandin E_2, 1-25-dihydroxyvitamin D, and mechanical forces
d. they are uninfluenced by parathyroid hormone or vitamin D levels

24-3. Osteoporosis is defined by a pathologic fracture, often in the spine, hip, or radial bones, or a DEXA scan with a T score of:

a. greater than or equal to 2.5
b. 0.1 to 2.5
c. −0.1 to −2.5
d. less than or equal to −2.5

24-4. Regarding treatment of osteoporosis

a. it should be treated with an increase in calcium and vitamin D intake and an exercise regimen
b. it should be treated with oral bisphosphonates such as Fosamax (alendronate)
c. it should be addressed hormonally
d. it should be individualized to the patient's needs and lifestyle in order to recreate balance and health for the patient

24-5. Which of the following are lab tests for bone formation?

a. urine hydroxyproline
b. serum bone specific alkaline phosphatase
c. urine deoxypyridinoline
d. urine hydroxylysine

24-6. Which of the following are lab tests for bone resorption?

a. serum procollagen I extension peptides
b. serum osteocalcin
c. urine pyridinoline
d. urine sodium

24-7. All of the following are true when considering calcium levels in a patient except

a. natural intake of calcium via food is superior to calcium supplements
b. calcium absorption requires an acidic stomach environment
c. calcium levels in bone are dependent on their ability to bind to the collagen matrix
d. medications do not alter calcium metabolism and absorption

24-8. Vitamin D is manufactured when sunlight alters the chemical structure of _____ in the skin.

a. cholesterol
b. estrogen
c. calcium
d. fatty acids

24-9. An individual with excess cortisol, either endogenous or exogenous, for a period of 3 months, will most likely not have any changes in bone mass density.

a. true
b. false

24-10. A 45-year-old female presents to your office with fibrocystic breast disease and complaints of foggy thinking, unexplained weight gain, increased PMS symptoms, insomnia, and water retention. What hormonal imbalance do you expect to find?

a. increased progesterone, increased estrogen
b. decreased progesterone, increased estrogen
c. increased progesterone, decreased estrogen
d. decreased progesterone, decreased estrogen

▶ CHAPTER 25. INTEGRATIVE APPROACH TO OTOLARYNGOLOGY

Learning Objectives:

a. describe three aspects of the integrative approach to treatment of recurrent otitis media in children
b. give three examples of the evidence regarding the use of herbal medicines in the treatment or prevention of recurrent upper respiratory infection
c. list three integrative therapeutic approaches to the treatment of sinusitis

25-1. What percentage of patients with asthma and sinusitis has reported using alternative medicine to manage their illness?

a. 33%
b. 42%
c. 56%
d. 78%

25-2. Echinacea has been proven effective as chemoprophylaxis for upper respiratory infections (URIs).

a. true
b. false

25-3. Vitamin C in high doses has been proven to be an effective chemoprophylactic agent against upper respiratory infections (URIs).

a. true
b. false

25-4. Up to _____% of acute otitis media will resolve without treatment.

a. 10%
b. 20%
c. 60%
d. 90%

25-5. Patients treated with homeopathic preparations tended to have all of the following except

a. earlier pain relief
b. shorter duration of therapy
c. fewer recurrences
d. less tympanic membrane perforations

25-6. The only side effect of xylitol gum when used for otitis media was

a. nausea
b. vomiting
c. diarrhea
d. rash

25-7. The proposed mechanism of action of osteopathy for otitis media includes all the following EXCEPT

a. lysis of adhesions around the eustachian tube
b. normalization of function of hyoid musculature
c. realignment of the fifth and eighth cranial nerves
d. lymphatic drainage

25-8. Hypertonic nasal saline irrigation is widely accepted as adjunctive treatment for sinusitis.

a. true
b. false

25-9. The Cleveland Clinic Study established that zinc gluconate lozenges are ineffective in the treatment of URIs.

a. true
b. false

25-10. All of the following are considered demulcents except

a. marshmallow leaf
b. marshmallow root
c. plantain
d. honeysuckle
e. *Astragalus*

▶ CHAPTER 26. INTEGRATIVE APPROACH TO PAIN

Learning Objectives:

a. discuss the evidence for the use of three botanical medicines and/or nutritional supplements in the treatment of pain syndromes
b. summarize the evidence for the use of mind–body approaches in patients with chronic pain
c. discuss the evidence for and against the use of acupuncture, chiropractic, and electromagnetic therapies in treatment of back pain

26-1. The JCAHO requires that pain be assessed and treated

a. on every H & P
b. only in the ambulatory care setting
c. as a vital sign
d. as ordered by the physician of record
e. when the patient complains of pain

26-2. The National Institutes of Health

a. has not yet looked into acupuncture

b. has not endorsed a multidisciplinary approach to pain

c. has found consensus that relaxation helps relieve pain

d. considers spinal manipulation helpful

e. is not currently researching CAM

26-3. Massage therapy for pain

a. may also improve insomnia

b. is covered by most insurance plans

c. has not been studied for workplace injuries

d. should not be used in fibromyalgia

e. probably does not last as long as acupuncture

26-4. There is good evidence that

a. Alexander work can cure back pain

b. yoga and massage work well together for arthritis

c. stagnation of QI can cause pain

d. Chinese medicine was not practiced in the United States before 1970

e. acupuncture can relieve nausea

26-5. Acupuncture

a. is inappropriate for postoperative patients

b. needles are only placed in points on the meridians

c. is not helpful in fibromyalgia

d. treatments are based on energetic patterns of diagnosis

e. is used to stop the flow of Qi

26-6. It is appropriate to

a. send a patient to a chiropractor three times a week for 3 months

b. send a rheumatoid arthritis patient to a chiropractor for cervical high velocity low amplitude manipulation (HVLA)

c. discourage a patient from chiropractic if a click is heard during treatment

d. always recommend osteopaths over chiropractors

e. recommend a trial of six to eight visits only to a chiropractor

26-7. Dietary supplements

a. containing minerals have no role in pain

b. containing omega-6 fatty acids increase the levels of arachidonic acid

c. containing leukotrienes can decrease pain

d. containing omega-3 fatty acids increase inflammation

e. containing borage oil are a source of omega-6 fatty acids

26-8. Glucosamine sulfate for the pain of osteoarthritis

a. has not been rigorously studied

b. may be helpful for knee degenerative joint disease (DJD)

c. is not as effective as shark cartilage

d. may work by the placebo effect

e. is free of side effects

26-9. Supplements for pain

a. can work as well as opioids

b. cannot have a dangerous reaction because they are natural

c. can raise blood pressure

d. should only be bought at health food stores

e. do not have recommended daily allowances

26-10. Nonionizing magnetic fields

a. always produce heat

b. have no effect on knee pain

c. may have effects on membrane transport

d. do not influence genetic expression

e. are not to be used with acupuncture points

▶ **CHAPTER 27. INTEGRATIVE APPROACH TO PULMONARY DISORDERS**

Learning Objectives:

a. give two examples of nutritional supplements shown to be useful in the treatment of asthma

b. discuss the role of dietary manipulation in the treatment of asthma and COPD

c. discuss the evidence for and against the use of acupuncture for asthma and COPD

27-1. Common causes of food sensitivity in children contributing to asthma symptoms include

a. wheat products
b. dairy products
c. aspartame
d. tartrazine
e. soy products

27-2. Meta-analysis has shown that breastfeeding can reduce the likelihood of developing asthma by 30–50% if it is continued for at least

a. 1 month
b. 3 months
c. 6 months
d. 1 year

27-3. Magnesium supplementation has been shown to be helpful in which of the following situations?

a. acute asthma
b. chronic asthma
c. both

27-4. Studies to date have shown chiropractic manipulation to be helpful in the management of asthma in adults but not in children.

a. true
b. false

27-5. *Boswellia serrata* is believed to have its effect in asthma via the action of boswellic acids. These compounds are purported to work as

a. beta-2 agonists
b. steroid potentiators
c. leukotriene antagonists
d. mucolytics

27-6. Herbs that have been shown at least potentially to have steroid-sparing effects in patients with asthma include

a. licorice
b. ma huang
c. lobelia
d. saiboku-tu
e. ginkgo

27-7. Vitamin C has been shown to be moderately effective in reducing airway hypersensitivity. Which of the following mechanisms have been proposed to explain this effect?

a. decreasing edema in the bronchial wall
b. antagonizing prostaglandin-induced bronchoconstriction
c. shifting leukotriene synthesis pathways from the five series to the four series
d. reducing oxidative stress in the airway

27-8. The air filtration technique that has shown some promise in reducing environmental triggers of asthma is

a. positive ion generation
b. high-efficiency particle filtration
c. positive pressure air filtration
d. ultraviolet air filtration

27-9. Which of the following food groups were associated with higher measures of FEV_1 in participants in the MORGEN study?

a. fruits
b. vegetables
c. whole grains
d. fish

27-10. Acupuncture has been shown to have no benefit either in subjective or objective measures of COPD.

a. true
b. false

▶ CHAPTER 28. INTEGRATIVE APPROACH TO PSYCHIATRY

Learning Objectives:

a. give three examples of the integrative approach to treatment of anxiety
b. summarize the evidence regarding the use of botanicals and nutritional supplements in the treatment of depression
c. give two examples of nutritional interventions that have been studied in the treatment of schizophrenia

28-1. Regarding the role of the doctor's attitude and expectations of patient responses to medication

a. the effect of physicians' attitudes toward drugs is minimal in explaining variance in drug effects
b. drug effects greater than placebo were observed among patients whose doctors expected a drug-placebo difference, but not among patients whose doctors were noncommittal
c. Uhlenhuth's experiment took place at Johns Hopkins University
d. b and c
e. all of the above

28-2. Regarding diet and depression

a. less anxiety and depression has been reported among vegetarians when compared to nonvegetarians
b. antioxidants can contribute to depression
c. slow weight reduction in overweight women is a risk factor for depression
d. eating breakfast regularly leads to improved mood, better memory, more energy, and feelings of calmness.
e. a and d

28-3. Regarding omega fatty acids

a. higher levels of fish consumption are associated with more depression and suicide among large populations
b. geographic areas where consumption of DHA is high are associated with decreased rates of depression
c. DHA-deficient states such as alcoholism and the postpartum period are also linked with depression
d. a and c
e. b and c

28-4. Regarding DHEA (dihydroepiandrosterone)

a. supplementation has not shown to be beneficial in some cases for major depression
b. positive effects on sexual interest and satisfaction and sense of well-being are more consistent in elderly women than in men
c. the recommended administered dose is 0.25–0.50 mg once a day in women and 1.0 mg in men
d. androgenic side effects (greasy skin, acne, increased growth of body hair) can occur and are irreversible
e. no risk exists for hormone-dependent cancer such as breast cancer in women and prostate cancer in men
f. screening for breast and prostate cancers before starting DHEA, as well as ongoing monitoring is not necessary

28-5. Regarding S-adenosylmethionine (SAMe)

a. SAMe is a synthetic substance that serves as a methyl donor and may contribute to an increase in the levels of certain neurotransmitters when given in supplement form

b. SAMe appears to have no antidepressant effect

c. SAMe appears to be well tolerated, with the majority of adverse effects presenting as mild to moderate gastrointestinal complaints

d. Di Rocco et al. reported a pilot study of SAMe in 13 depressed patients with Addison disease

e. SAMe was administered in doses of 80–360 mg per day for a period of 10 weeks

28-6. Valerian root

a. is used as an antianxiety agent, but does not have antidepressant and sedative properties

b. is not indicated for long-term treatment of sleep disorders

c. improves the sleep of insomniacs after benzodiazepine withdrawal

d. is not effective in stress symptoms and stress-related insomnia

e. a, b, and c

28-7. Aerobic exercise

a. does not reduce anxiety

b. decreases somatic symptoms of anxiety, but leaves cognitive/anxiety symptoms (mental and emotional) unchanged

c. decreased psychological symptoms of anxiety with unchanged somatic symptoms

d. reduces anxiety but not depression

e. has effects that wear off over time, even with continuing participation in regular exercise

28-8. Movement therapies

a. Tai Chi participation reduces anxiety

b. compared to controls, men in a Tai Chi group experienced significant reductions in anxiety, depression, anger, confusion, total mood disturbance, and improved general mood

c. women did not have significant results

d. a and b

e. a and c

28-9. Regarding relaxation/meditation

a. it has been shown to reduce anxiety and improve depression

b. a program consisting of a 2-hour weekly class for 8 weeks in training and experiencing mindful meditation is sufficient to see improvements in anxiety and depression (with a one-time 7.5-hour intensive silent meditation retreat in the sixth week)

c. panic symptoms do not improve

d. agoraphobia indices do not improve

e. a and b

28-10. Regarding biofeedback

a. the usefulness of biofeedback in the treatment of anxiety disorders has never been statistically demonstrated

b. nine weekly thermal biofeedback sessions with home BP monitoring is sufficient to lower SBP, DBP, heart rate, and cardiac output

c. differences were not maintained 3 years afterwards

d. reduces urinary cortisol and aldosterone

e. b and d

▶ CHAPTER 29. INTEGRATIVE APPROACH TO RHEUMATOLOGY

Learning Objectives:

a. give three examples of integrative therapeutic approaches to rheumatoid arthritis

b. discuss the use of botanicals and nutritional supplements in the treatment of osteoarthritis

c. discuss and give three examples of integrative approaches that may be helpful in the treatment of fibromyalgia

29-1. Which of the following should be avoided in patients with gout?

a. alcoholic beverages
b. nonsteroidal anti-inflammatory medications
c. increased water intake
d. dark berries

29-2. Which of the following methods has not been shown to be helpful in fibromyalgia in controlled trials?

a. nonsteroidal antiinflammatory medications
b. tricyclic antidepressants
c. *Chorella pyrenoidosa*
d. *Rhus toxicodendron* 6c

29-3. Studies have shown that despite treatment, this percentage of patients with fibromyalgia continue to show symptoms 2–5 years after diagnosis

a. 0–10%
b. 10–20%
c. 20–45%
d. 45–100%

29-4. Glucosamine sulfate is considered this type of agent

a. a nonsteroidal antiinflammatory drug
b. a structure-modifying agent
c. a symptom-modifying agent
d. a steroid

29-5. Using an elimination diet to see if a particular food group worsens symptoms in a patient with rheumatoid arthritis (RA).

a. is not as good as serum testing, which is the gold standard
b. is worthless because food has no effect on RA symptoms
c. is easy for the patient to perform with excellent compliance rates
d. can be both diagnostic and therapeutic

29-6. Which is *not* true regarding using fasting for therapeutic benefit in rheumatoid arthritis?

a. fasting has been found to reduce inflammatory markers such as C-reactive protein and interleukin-6
b. fasting has been shown to induce prolonged remission in autoimmune disease
c. benefits of fasting provide support that certain foods may trigger inflammatory changes
d. there is no need to monitor electrolytes if fasting is used for more than 5 days

29-7. Coffee in amounts greater than four cups a day has been associated with a higher risk of developing rheumatoid arthritis.

a. true
b. false

29-8. Gamma-linoleic acid (GLA)

a. is an omega-3 fatty acid
b. is an omega-6 fatty acid and a source of arachidonic acid
c. has not been found to be of any benefit in rheumatoid arthritis
d. is found in large amounts in borage oil, black current oil, flax seed oil, and cold-water fish

29-9. Journaling to express emotions that may be related to physical symptoms

a. has been found to reduce rheumatoid arthritis symptoms by 28% in one well done study
b. is without any potential side effects
c. is simply the process of writing down what you did during the day
d. is subject to economic bias due to the high profit margins of paper and pencils

29-10. Acupuncture for osteoarthritis pain

a. is no better than placebo
b. reduces pain as much as NSAIDs, but long-term effects need further study
c. has been found to increase the risk of a septic joint
d. improves both knee pain and function

▶ CHAPTER 30. INTEGRATIVE APPROACH TO THE CARE OF CHILDREN: WELL-CHILD CARE

Learning Objectives:

a. discuss the evidence for and against the safety of co-sleeping and for and against the safety of home birth
b. list three measures parents can take to reduce a child's exposure to environmental hazards
c. discuss three of the most common concerns parents raise regarding childhood vaccinations and the evidence regarding vaccine safety

30-1. The following factors are critical in ensuring a low rate of adverse outcomes in out-of-hospital births

a. excluding twins
b. presence of a trained birth attendant
c. excluding first pregnancies
d. excluding postdates pregnancies

30-2. The practice of continuous fetal monitoring in hospital births has been shown to contribute to which of the following?

a. lower rates of neurologic birth-related deficits
b. higher rates of cesarean section
c. decreased rates of maternal hemorrhage

30-3. The incidence of SIDS appears to be higher in co-sleeping families if

a. the mother is a smoker
b. the infant was premature
c. the child is not breastfeeding
d. the child sleeps between parents rather than at the edge of the bed

30-4. The most important role of fluoride in preventing tooth decay appears to be

a. prior to baby tooth eruption
b. following baby tooth eruption
c. following permanent tooth eruption

30-5. The NAHMES II health survey found a significantly increased percentage of body fat and increased BMI in children watching how many hours of television per day?

a. greater than 1
b. 2–4
c. greater than 4

30-6. There are homeopathic vaccination protocols that have been shown to be effective in preliminary trials for a number of childhood diseases.

a. true
b. false

30-7. The Institute of Medicine reports from 1991 and 1994 concluded that out of 76 vaccine adverse reactions they reviewed, what percentage had adequate data to draw definitive conclusions about safety?

a. 10%
b. 34%
c. 70%

30-8. Standard single-dose childhood immunizations contain thimerosal, a mercury-based preservative.

a. true
b. false

30-9. Exposure to PCBs in utero has been shown to be associated with which of the following?

a. lower IQ scores
b. increased rates of childhood cancers
c. increased rates of liver disease
d. decreased reading comprehension

30-10. The following fish are potentially extremely high in mercury

a. swordfish
b. sardines
c. cod
d. fresh tuna

▶ CHAPTER 31. INTEGRATIVE APPROACH TO COMMON PEDIATRIC CONDITIONS

Learning Objectives:

a. describe three dimensions of the integrative approach to atopic dermatitis
b. discuss the use of supplements and botanicals in the treatment of acne
c. summarize the nutritional approaches currently popular for the treatment of autism

31-1. Which of the following about zinc is true?

a. zinc has been consistently proven to be helpful in the treatment of acne
b. the appropriate initial dose of zinc for acne is 30 mg bid–tid
c. zinc takes about 4 months to show efficacy for acne
d. prolonged intake of zinc can cause iron deficiency

31-2. Regarding nutritional therapies for autism

a. meat and sugar are most commonly eliminated to improve autism
b. the basis for the gluten/casein free diet is the opioid theory of autism
c. in the urine of almost all people with autism there appear to be elevated levels of substances with properties similar to those expected from opioid peptides
d. defective intestinal enzymes (especially dipeptidyl-dipeptidase IV) allow incompletely digested meat proteins to "leak" across the gut and into the bloodstream
e. a and d

31-3. Regarding pyridoxine (vitamin B_6 in autism)

a. vitamin B_6, or pyridoxine, plays a key role in the synthesis of certain neurotransmitters
b. the risks of supplementation with high-dose vitamin B_6 and magnesium consist of physical aggression and decreased social responsiveness
c. doses of B_6 range from 1.5–3.0 mg per kilogram of body weight per day (70–100 mg/day)
d. the majority of studies combine B_6 with copper

31-4. Regarding the role of environmental toxins in autism

a. the argument that links autism to environmental toxins draws upon extensive studies of the role of environmental toxins including pesticides and herbicides in the pathogenesis of autism
b. proponents of the environmental toxin theory argue that early exposure to synthetic chemicals is one possible explanation for the recent dramatic increase in the incidence of autism
c. children with autism show normal liver detoxification profiles
d. children with autism show increased levels of toxic chemicals, often exceeding adult maximum tolerance
e. b and d

31-5. Regarding touch therapy for autism

a. massage therapy is more effective than a reading attention control group
b. changes occurred, primarily a reduction in violent behavior
c. massage therapy has resulted in lower anxiety and stress hormones and improved clinical course
d. grandparent or parent volunteers are not as helpful as professionals
e. a and c

31-6. Concerning the role of food allergy in atopic dermatitis (AD), all of the following statements are correct except

a. recent studies have confirmed that food allergy plays a role in many patients with AD
b. the double-blind placebo-controlled food challenge (DBPCFC) is considered the gold standard for research in food allergy
c. this is because the DBPCFC has excellent sensitivity and specificity for both immediate and delayed food reactions
d. neither skin prick testing nor food-specific IGE (i.e., RAST) can be relied upon to diagnose or rule out food allergy

31-7. Which of the following are among the most common food allergens?

a. egg, milk, wheat, avocado, and fish
b. egg, strawberries, wheat, fish, and nuts
c. egg, dairy, wheat, fish, soy, and nuts
d. dairy, wheat, peanuts, strawberries, and pineapple

31-8. Concerning probiotics for the prevention of AD, all of the following are true except

a. probiotics given to pregnant and breastfeeding mothers have been shown to decrease the incidence of eczema in their babies at age 2 years
b. it is not safe to give infants probiotic supplements in their formula
c. the presumed mechanism of action of probiotics is immunoprotection through alteration of gut flora
d. studies generally indicate that probiotics for the prevention of AD work best when given to families with a high genetic risk for atrophy

31-9. Breast-feeding has definitely been proven to help prevent atopic dermatitis.

a. true
b. false

31-10. Which two of the following statements are true concerning mind–body therapies for AD?

a. there are a number of randomized controlled studies demonstrating the efficacy of these treatments for AD
b. if they are helpful, it is only through reducing anxiety and scratching
c. modalities like hypnosis or biofeedback can influence the autonomic nervous system, resulting in endocrine or immune responses that can directly affect the pathophysiological mechanisms of AD
d. a number of noncontrolled trials have shown these modalities to be helpful for the treatment of AD
e. a and b
f. c and d

▶ CHAPTER 32. INTEGRATIVE APPROACH TO PREGNANCY

Learning Objectives:

a. list three examples of integrative approaches to pregnancy-related symptoms or complaints

b. discuss the safety issues pertaining to the use of Chinese medicine, massage, aromatic oils, and homeopathy in pregnancy, and list one possible safe use of each of these therapies

c. list three herbs contraindicated in pregnancy and lactation

32-1. Acupuncture at pericardium-6 (P-6), or the Neiguan point, has shown efficacy for the treatment of what discomforts of pregnancy?

a. insomnia
b. heartburn
c. nausea and vomiting

32-2. The two substances that have demonstrated the greatest efficacy in clinical trials for the treatment of morning sickness are

a. progesterone and estrogen
b. vitamin B_6 and ginger
c. echinacea and cramp bark

32-3. Chinese herbs should be used with extreme caution during pregnancy because

a. they are well known to contain botanical substitutions, adulterants, heavy metals, and added pharmaceuticals frequently not listed on the label, all of which can pose threat to the safety of the pregnant woman and fetus
b. their import into the United States is entirely unregulated
c. Chinese herbs should only be used in combination with other Chinese herbs

32-4. Numerous studies on the use of homeopathic medicines during pregnancy have demonstrated

a. great efficacy in the treatment of many common complaints of pregnancy
b. little that is conclusive due to poor studies, small sample sizes, and research methodologies that are inconsistent with the principles upon which homeopathy is based
c. that *Caulophyllum thalictroides* is highly effective at stimulating the onset of labor

32-5. Exposure to essential oils has led to the initiation of seizures, hypertension, hypotension, photosensitivity, and abortion.

a. true
b. false

32-6. A generally safe approach to using essential oils during pregnancy is to

a. use essential oils externally only, and in a dilute form
b. dilute essential oils well in water before consuming
c. use concentrated and undiluted essential oils for serious health conditions only

32-7. Emmenagogues are herbs and oils that may

a. be used safely during the first trimester of pregnancy
b. enhance lactation
c. cause commencement of the menses or general uterine bleeding

32-8. During the first trimester of pregnancy it is *preferable* to

a. entirely avoid the use of herbs if possible
b. avoid the use of mutagenic and teratogenic herbs only
c. use herbs freely as long as they are not contraindicated during pregnancy

32-9. Echinacea, which has been demonstrated in recent clinical trials to be safe for use during pregnancy, is most effective when used

a. in large and frequent doses
b. in small and frequent doses
c. in large and infrequent doses

32-10. Blue cohosh, a common herb for stimulating labor, is a safe and reliable herb to use in late pregnancy to tone the uterus.

a. true
b. false

▶ **CHAPTER 33. INTEGRATIVE APPROACH TO COMMON CONDITIONS IN WOMEN'S HEALTH**

Learning Objectives:

a. list three herbal medicines often useful in the treatment of vaginitis

b. discuss and give examples of three of the integrative therapeutic approaches to PMS for which reasonable evidence of efficacy is available

c. give three examples of integrative approaches to the treatment of fibroids

33-1. Studies suggest that women with PMS typically consume diets that are higher in the following

a. dairy products
b. refined sugar
c. caffeinated beverages
d. b and c
e. all of the above

33-2. A systematic review of the efficacy of vitamin B_6 in women with PMS suggests that benefit may be achieved from B_6 supplementation at a dose of 250 mg/day and may even result in improvement of depressive symptoms.

a. true
b. false

33-3. Black cohosh (*Cimicifuga racemosa*)

a. appears to act by suppressing both LH and FSH levels
b. has been shown to benefit various menopausal symptoms (hot flashes, profuse sweating, sleep disturbance, and depressive moods) that are also present in women with PMS
c. a only
d. b only
e. a and b

33-4. Regular, moderate aerobic exercise appears to offer effective improvement of impaired concentration, negative affect, behavior change, and pain in women with PMS.

a. true
b. false

33-5. The mainstay of treatment in vaginitis is

a. to restore the natural balance of the body and remove the offending source
b. immediately start antibiotics or antimycotics
c. add high protein to the diet
d. eliminate sexual contact

33-6. Botanicals used in the treatment of candidal vaginitis include

a. garlic
b. feverfew
c. tea tree oil
d. milk thistle

33-7. Plants with phytoestrogen activity include

a. black cohosh
b. garlic
c. licorice
d. red clover

33-8. A study of a combination of traditional Chinese medicine, pelvic bodywork, and guided imagery training versus conventional treatment of fibroids showed these statistically significant results

a. more satisfaction with treatment in the integrative medicine group

b. more fibroid shrinkage or cessation of growth in the integrative medicine group

c. more decrease in symptoms in the integrative medicine group

33-9. A diet rich in phytoestrogens may be protective against uterine fibroids by

a. competing with endogenous estrogens and influencing sex hormone production

b. increasing plasma estrogen levels and decreasing fecal estrogen excretion

c. decreasing plasma estrogen levels as a result of increased fiber in such a diet

33-10. Randomized controlled trials show a statistically significant effect of the following modalities in the treatment of uterine fibroids

a. homeopathy

b. chiropractic

c. Ayurveda

d. exercise

e. all of the above

f. none of the above

▶ CHAPTER 34. INTEGRATIVE APPROACH TO MENOPAUSE

Learning Objectives:

a. discuss the use of botanicals and phytoestrogens for symptoms of menopause

b. discuss the current evidence regarding the connection between hormone replacement therapy and the risks of breast and ovarian cancer

c. discuss the pros and cons of bioidentical versus standard hormone replacement

34-1. Which of the following is true?

a. the only mechanism by which estrogen and phytoestrogens exert actions on tissues is through estrogen receptor binding

b. after 5–6 months of complete amenorrhea, you can reliably inform your patient that she is menopausal and no longer fertile

c. the perimenopause may last longer than 5 years

d. the onset of menopause is the only reason a 50-year-old previously menstruating woman would cease to menstruate for more than a few months

34-2. All of the following are false except

a. salivary testing for estrogen is a reliable, validated method for measuring estrogen levels in perimenopausal women

b. accurate steady-state blood estrogen levels can be obtained 72 hours after a change in estrogen dosage

c. you know your patient is receiving adequate estrogen dosing when the FSH level during treatment is driven back into the reproductive age-range level for your reference lab

d. progestins have minimal effect on sex hormone-binding globulin (SHBG) levels, while estrogen and thyroid hormone increase them

e. there appears to be an accurate correlation between blood and salivary levels of testosterone during treatment and salivary levels and clinical responses to treatment in women

34-3. Which of the following is true?

A. unlike estrogen levels, salivary progesterone levels are generally reliable to monitor treatment, especially from transdermal administration

B. salivary measurement of growth hormone and DHEA have shown reliable correlation with serum measurement for diagnosis and monitoring of related conditions

a. A

b. B

c. both

d. neither

34-4. Which of the following is true?

a. if your perimenopausal or menopausal patient is having problems with insomnia, estrogen supplementation alone should fix the problem, so there is no need for further inquiry or education

b. short-term prescription of pharmaceutical sleep agents should be your first treatment choice for a menopausal patient that comes to you complaining of difficulty sleeping

c. before prescribing medication for sleep disturbances, it is reasonable to screen her for the use of precipitating drugs, medications, or alcohol and make an assessment of her sleep hygiene with education and/or references provided as needed

d. since standardized valerian root capsules are so safe, any patient can use them every night over extended periods of time if she feels she needs them

e. guided imagery and hypnotherapy have been proven unhelpful for the treatment of insomnia

34-5. All of the following are true except

a. there are associations between dietary intake, inflammation, and the development of chronic disease

b. support of optimal liver metabolism and improved inhibition of reabsorption of metabolized estrogen into the bowel lumen with adequate intake of fiber will help minimize excessive levels of circulating estrogens in the blood

c. it is fine to take daily calcium supplements at the same time of day as acid suppressant medications

d. purees and juices of fruits and vegetables are excellent ways to palatably increase the number of daily servings in our diets

e. drinking ice-cold drinks before or with meals diminishes digestive efficiency

34-6. Which of the following is true regarding botanicals?

A. if your patient uses a botanical for a week and gets no response, she can be assured that it won't work for her

B. some botanicals may take up to 12 weeks of continuous use for the full response to be realized

C. evening primrose oil may be effective for the treatment of cyclic mastalgia

D. topical Mexican yam cream has been proven in double-blind placebo-controlled crossover studies to be very effective for the treatment of menopausal symptoms

E. black cohosh (*Cimicifuga racemosa*) is the only botanical proven in well-designed clinical studies to be effective for vasomotor symptoms, sweating, headaches, vertigo, palpitations, and sleep disturbances associated with the menopause

a. A and D

b. A, B, and C

c. B, D, and F

d. B, C, E, and F

e. B, C, and E

34-7. Which one of the following statements regarding phytoestrogens is false?

a. phytoestrogens have structures very similar to estrogens and have no antiestrogenic actions under any circumstances

b. different phytoestrogens have different percentages of isoflavones, which is the component found to have the most potent estrogenic activity as compared to all other phytoestrogen components

c. isoflavones bind preferentially to ER-beta receptors so they express their estrogenic activities in CNS, blood vessels, bone, and skin without stimulating the uterus or breast in vitro

d. the major soy isoflavones are genistein and daidzein

e. studies have shown that soy isoflavones may be helpful for the reduction of hot flush frequency

f. until the safety issues surrounding the dosage of high-dose isoflavone products are further elucidated, it is prudent to recommend dietary isoflavone sources for your patients, and if they do use isolated isoflavone supplements, to avoid taking more than 100 mg per day

34-8. Which of the following is true?

a. bioidentical hormones are those that are chemically indistinguishable from the hormones produced by the human body

b. Premarin is not a natural-sourced estrogen product

c. plant-sourced natural products can be used by humans directly without any further chemical modification

d. estriol, the weakest of all the circulating estrogens, has been proven to have no estrogenic effect on the endometrium, myometrium, or vagina and so may be used as a supplement safely, without concurrent progesterone, in a woman with a uterus in situ

34-9. Which of the following is false?

a. the vast majority of studies on the potential effects (beneficial or adverse) of hormones, especially with respect to chronic disease prevention, have used oral conjugated equine estrogen

b. the vast majority of studies regarding the potential effects of using hormone supplementation therapy have used a wide variety of estrogen preparations

c. the "first-pass effect" of oral estrogens includes enhancement of the production of binding globulins, triglycerides, clotting factors, and HDL-cholesterol (among others). Transdermal estrogens, as they first exert actions before they reach the liver, do not cause these same effects, or at least not to a degree that is clinically significant

d. oral bioidentical micronized progesterone has less of a blunting effect on the beneficial effects of estrogen on serum lipids and carbohydrate metabolism than synthetic progestins

34-10. Which of the following is true?

A. data from earlier large observational epidemiologic studies such as the Nurses Health Study suggested that estrogen replacement was effective for the prevention and treatment of some chronic diseases such as heart disease

B. every woman with a uterus who is prescribed estrogen therapy requires concurrent progestin supplementation to stabilize the endometrium and prevent the unopposed estrogen-induced endometrial hyperplasia and endometrial adenocarcinoma. For those unable to tolerate *any* form of oral progesterone, other routes of administration are available

C. absolute contraindications of estrogen therapy include history of thrombotic disease, serious or current liver disease, undiagnosed genitourinary bleeding, suspected pregnancy, and suspicion of an estrogen dependent cancer

a. A only
b. B only
c. C only
d. all
e. none

▶ CHAPTER 35. INTEGRATIVE APPROACH TO GERIATRICS

Learning Objectives:

a. list three benefits of tai chi in the elderly for which significant research evidence exists

b. discuss the potential role of spiritual issues in the health of the elderly

c. list three herbs that may be helpful in common problems in the elderly and discuss any contraindications that exist for each

35-1. Pick the correct answer

a. nearly one-half of elderly individuals over the age of 65 fall each year
b. of those who reach age 80, approximately 50% will fall in a given year
c. of those who reach 80, half fall repeatedly
d. at least 10% of older people suffer serious injuries due to falls
e. b and d

35-2. Which of the following are included in the "SCOPED" mnemonic for geriatric care?

a. SAFETY (is the patient at risk for accidents?)
b. COUNT (can the patient handle money?)
c. OPERATE A CAR (ask about driving accidents and incidents; consider driving evaluation)
d. EXECUTIVE FUNCTIONS (exercise good judgment)
e. a, b, and c
f. all of the above

35-3. *Ginkgo biloba* does not prevent cerebral ischemia and transient ischemic attacks.

a. true
b. false

35-4. Mark the correct answer

a. Qigong has not actually been shown to lower blood pressure
b. Qigong increases social interaction and builds self-confidence
c. Qigong emphasizes repetitive patterns of moving
d. a and b
e. b and c

35-5. Regarding studies comparing oxazepam and valerian, pick what is true

a. 202 outpatients aged 18 to 73 years and diagnosed with nonorganic insomnia according to ICD-10 (F 51.0) were treated in a multicenter double-blind, randomized parallel group comparison with either 600 mg/day valerian extract LI 156 (Sedonium) or 10 mg/day oxazepam taken for 6 weeks
b. mean duration of insomnia was 1 year at baseline
c. valerian was equivalent to oxazepam
d. all of the above
e. b and c

35-6. Regarding nutrition and vision, select the correct answers

a. higher intake of carotenoids, including lutein and zeaxanthin (found in dark green leafy vegetables such as spinach and collard greens) is helpful
b. increased intake of protein can be helpful
c. combinations of antioxidants, including 600 mg selenium, 1.2 g vitamin E, 80 mg vitamin B_6, 15 mg vitamin B_2, and 2 g vitamin C daily for 5 months are useful
d. multivitamins did not further reduce the risk in one study but did in another
e. a, c, and d

35-7. Regarding the prevention of osteoporosis

a. increasing grains can be helpful as can reducing the amount of sodium in the diet
b. increasing magnesium is important, as is reducing protein intake
c. increasing phosphoric acid is helpful
d. diagnosing and treating celiac disease (which increases fat-soluble minerals and vitamins, especially calcium and vitamin D) is helpful
e. b and d

35-8. Further steps to prevent osteoporosis include

a. avoiding nicotine and vitamin D
b. walking and jogging
c. calcium supplementation, and generally all calcium preparations are equally good
d. taking trace minerals
e. b and d

35-9. Regarding niacinamide in the treatment of osteoarthritis

a. 72 patients with osteoarthritis were treated with 500 mg of niacinamide six times daily for 12 weeks or with a placebo in double-blind fashion
b. in the niacinamide group, global arthritis impact improved 59%
c. joint mobility increased by 4.5%
d. a and c
e. all of the above

35-10. For cancer patients, combination therapy with Qigong did not reduce the side effects of cancer therapy.

a. true
b. false

▶ CHAPTER 36. LEGAL AND ETHICAL ISSUES IN INTEGRATIVE MEDICINE

Learning Objectives:

a. list three strategies via which an integrative physician can minimize the risk of malpractice liability

b. give three examples of complications that may arise for a physician with practitioners of other healing arts working in the same office setting

c. summarize the current status of state regulation of integrative medical practice

36-1. The protection physicians obtain against malpractice actions by signed informed consent forms primarily arises because the form shows that

a. the physician and patient discussed the therapy
b. the patient assumed the risk of the potential adverse reactions listed on the form
c. the patient was exercising their Constitutional right to choose a therapy
d. the staff is conscientiously working at good patient communication

36-2. A chiropractor's risk of loss to a malpractice action is

a. higher than that of a medical physician
b. about the same as that of a physician
c. about one-quarter that of a physician
d. about one-tenth that of a physician

36-3. As a physician adopts CAM methods in their practice, he or she should do the following with regard to malpractice coverage

a. nothing; adding a CAM procedure is no different than adding any other developing therapy
b. give notice to the malpractice insurance carrier about any significant therapies that are added to the practice
c. get an additional policy rider that specifically covers integrative/CAM practices
d. start protecting their assets, as their carrier is unlikely to provide coverage

36-4. From a legal perspective, of the following, the most critical issue that integrative physicians and their patients need to be clear about is

a. the amount and type of training the physician has in integrative medicine
b. whether the role of the physician is as a primary care doctor, medical specialist, or simply delivering particular CAM therapies
c. what the patient's beliefs are about CAM
d. whether the patient has previously sued any practitioner

36-5. When documenting an alternative treatment in the medical record, it is most important that the physician make sure that he or she

a. focuses entirely on the basis for the treatment from a CAM perspective, to make sure that what he or she is doing is fully explained from that perspective
b. note that the patient insisted on using CAM
c. make sure that basic medical evaluation and consideration of possible conventional treatments are documented to make it clear that good medical practice was part of the consideration
d. document as little as possible in order to minimize the paper trail about CAM services

36-6. If a manufacturer wanted to make a legal claim about calcium and its impact on bone function, which of the following would be acceptable

a. "prevents or relieves osteoporosis"
b. "prevents bone fragility in postmenopausal women"
c. "helps build healthy bones"
d. "works with HRT to promote healthy bones in women"

36-7. The Federation of State Medical Boards suggested policy on physician sale of dietary supplements is

a. just like physician sales of dermatologic creams or orthopedic splints, it should be allowed
b. physicians should only sell brands that are assayed and show certified amounts of the active alkaloids
c. physicians should hire a certified pharmacist or other expert in herbal medicine to be on-site if such sales are to be made
d. physicians should not sell supplements as their self-interest in earning a profit creates a conflict of interest

36-8. Credentialing programs for integrative practice

a. include programs recognized by the American Board of Medical Specialties
b. include a variety of broad-based programs and certifications for specific CAM techniques that have varying degrees of credibility
c. have no value as they are not recognized by the American Board of Medical Specialties
d. have no real purpose as integrative medicine is really a philosophy

36-9. Privileging for services in a hospital means

a. assuring that a practitioner has the competence to practice in their field
b. assuring that a practitioner has the competence to practice the specific technique being privileged
c. assuring that a practitioner does not have adverse professional findings for negligence or disciplinary actions
d. none of the above

36-10. The best practical clinical protection against problems with hospital patient use of herbal products is

a. physician access to a good up-to-date database about herb–drug interactions
b. providing consultations between the patient and an herbal specialist
c. requiring all herbs to be purchased from the hospital pharmacy
d. a firm policy barring any patient use of herbs in the hospital

NOTES:

NOTES:

NOTES:

NOTES:

NOTES:

NOTES:

NOTES:

NOTES:

NOTES:

NOTES:

NOTES:

NOTES:

CME EVALUATION
QUESTIONNAIRE
& ANSWER SHEET

*This CME test is for the chapters indicated published in **Integrative Medicine CME Study Guide** and has been provided by InnoVision Communications. InnoVision Communications is accredited by the Accreditation Council for Continuing Medical Education to provide continuing medical education for physicians. InnoVision Communication designates this educational activity on an hour-for-hour basis toward category 1 credit of the AMA Physician Recognition Award. Each physician should only claim those hours of credit he/she actually spent in the educational activity.*

PLEASE PRINT

Name _____   Credentials _____

E-mail _____ Phone _____

Address _____

City _____ State _____ Zip Code _____ Country _____

No. Chapters completed (*Note: fee is $10 / chapter*)
_____

Credit Card Number _____   Card Expiration Date _____

Signature _____   Date _____

Please list your primary objective for partaking in this activity. _____
_____

Please list the primary benefits you received from this CME activity. _____
_____

What topics would you like to see addressed in future CME activities? _____
_____

Mail this Answer Sheet with your $10 payment/chapter to:
CME – InnoVision Communications
169 Saxony Road, Suite 103 – Encinitas, CA 92024

Please circle your answer.

Chapter # _____

Title _____

1	A	B	C	D	E	F
2	A	B	C	D	E	F
3	A	B	C	D	E	F
4	A	B	C	D	E	F
5	A	B	C	D	E	F
6	A	B	C	D	E	F
7	A	B	C	D	E	F
8	A	B	C	D	E	F
9	A	B	C	D	E	F
10	A	B	C	D	E	F

Chapter # _____

Title _____

1	A	B	C	D	E	F
2	A	B	C	D	E	F
3	A	B	C	D	E	F
4	A	B	C	D	E	F
5	A	B	C	D	E	F
6	A	B	C	D	E	F
7	A	B	C	D	E	F
8	A	B	C	D	E	F
9	A	B	C	D	E	F
10	A	B	C	D	E	F

Chapter # _____

Title _____

1	A	B	C	D	E	F
2	A	B	C	D	E	F
3	A	B	C	D	E	F
4	A	B	C	D	E	F
5	A	B	C	D	E	F
6	A	B	C	D	E	F
7	A	B	C	D	E	F
8	A	B	C	D	E	F
9	A	B	C	D	E	F
10	A	B	C	D	E	F

Chapter # _____

Title _____

1	A	B	C	D	E	F
2	A	B	C	D	E	F
3	A	B	C	D	E	F
4	A	B	C	D	E	F
5	A	B	C	D	E	F
6	A	B	C	D	E	F
7	A	B	C	D	E	F
8	A	B	C	D	E	F
9	A	B	C	D	E	F
10	A	B	C	D	E	F

Chapter # _____

Title _____

1	A	B	C	D	E	F
2	A	B	C	D	E	F
3	A	B	C	D	E	F
4	A	B	C	D	E	F
5	A	B	C	D	E	F
6	A	B	C	D	E	F
7	A	B	C	D	E	F
8	A	B	C	D	E	F
9	A	B	C	D	E	F
10	A	B	C	D	E	F

Chapter # _____

Title _____

1	A	B	C	D	E	F
2	A	B	C	D	E	F
3	A	B	C	D	E	F
4	A	B	C	D	E	F
5	A	B	C	D	E	F
6	A	B	C	D	E	F
7	A	B	C	D	E	F
8	A	B	C	D	E	F
9	A	B	C	D	E	F
10	A	B	C	D	E	F

Chapter # _____

Title _____

1	A	B	C	D	E	F
2	A	B	C	D	E	F
3	A	B	C	D	E	F
4	A	B	C	D	E	F
5	A	B	C	D	E	F
6	A	B	C	D	E	F
7	A	B	C	D	E	F
8	A	B	C	D	E	F
9	A	B	C	D	E	F
10	A	B	C	D	E	F

Chapter # _____

Title _____

1	A	B	C	D	E	F
2	A	B	C	D	E	F
3	A	B	C	D	E	F
4	A	B	C	D	E	F
5	A	B	C	D	E	F
6	A	B	C	D	E	F
7	A	B	C	D	E	F
8	A	B	C	D	E	F
9	A	B	C	D	E	F
10	A	B	C	D	E	F

Chapter # _____

Title _____

1	A	B	C	D	E	F
2	A	B	C	D	E	F
3	A	B	C	D	E	F
4	A	B	C	D	E	F
5	A	B	C	D	E	F
6	A	B	C	D	E	F
7	A	B	C	D	E	F
8	A	B	C	D	E	F
9	A	B	C	D	E	F
10	A	B	C	D	E	F

Chapter # _____

Title _____

1	A	B	C	D	E	F
2	A	B	C	D	E	F
3	A	B	C	D	E	F
4	A	B	C	D	E	F
5	A	B	C	D	E	F
6	A	B	C	D	E	F
7	A	B	C	D	E	F
8	A	B	C	D	E	F
9	A	B	C	D	E	F
10	A	B	C	D	E	F

Chapter # _____

Title _____

1	A	B	C	D	E	F
2	A	B	C	D	E	F
3	A	B	C	D	E	F
4	A	B	C	D	E	F
5	A	B	C	D	E	F
6	A	B	C	D	E	F
7	A	B	C	D	E	F
8	A	B	C	D	E	F
9	A	B	C	D	E	F
10	A	B	C	D	E	F

Chapter # _____

Title _____

1	A	B	C	D	E	F
2	A	B	C	D	E	F
3	A	B	C	D	E	F
4	A	B	C	D	E	F
5	A	B	C	D	E	F
6	A	B	C	D	E	F
7	A	B	C	D	E	F
8	A	B	C	D	E	F
9	A	B	C	D	E	F
10	A	B	C	D	E	F